50 THINGS

EVERY

Young Lady

SHOULD KNOW

50 THINGS

EVERY

Young Lady

SHOULD KNOW

WHAT TO DO,
WHAT TO SAY,
AND HOW TO BEHAVE

KAY WEST
with JOHN BRIDGES
and BRYAN CURTIS

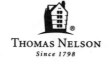

Thomas Nelson
Since 1798

NASHVILLE   DALLAS   MEXICO CITY   RIO DE JANEIRO

Published in Nashville, Tennessee, by Thomas Nelson. Thomas Nelson is a registered trademark of Thomas Nelson, Inc.

Thomas Nelson, Inc., titles may be purchased in bulk for educational, business, fund-raising, or sales promotional use. For information, please e-mail SpecialMarkets@ThomasNelson.com.

ISBN: 978-14041-83513 (BB)

Library of Congress Cataloging-in-Publication Data

West, Kay, 1955–
  50 things every young lady should know : what to do, when to do it, and why / Kay West with John Bridges and Bryan Curtis.
     p. cm.
  Includes bibliographical references and index.
  ISBN 978-1-4016-0064-8 (alk. paper)
  1. Etiquette for girls. 2. Etiquette for children and teenagers. I. Bridges, John, 1950– II. Curtis, Bryan, 1960– III. Title. IV. Title: Fifty things every young lady should know.
  BJ1857.G5W47 2011
  395.1'233—dc23

2011017949

Printed in the United States of America

12 13 14 15 WOR 6

To my mother,
Joyce Karlson Shaw,
who laid the foundation, and to her sister
Donalyn Karlson Morris,
who let me tag along

—K.W.

CONTENTS

INTRODUCTION

*I*t's safe to say that young women in the 21st century are exposed to more educational opportunities than any generation of women in history. Even before you started kindergarten you might have been on a soccer team, in a dance class, or taking Suzuki violin lessons. At home you might have played word games on the computer and practiced writing your name. By the time you get to middle school, you might feel as if there aren't enough hours in the week to do everything on your calendar.

But sometimes what gets lost in between ballet and biology, Spanish class and piano lessons, creative writing and cross country, are the basic rules of simple etiquette and guidelines for appropriate behavior.

Years and years ago, young ladies were expected to take classes in proper deportment, which is an old-fashioned way of saying simple etiquette and appropriate behavior. That was long before young women spent their teen years preparing for higher education, interesting work, and being financially independent.

Progress is a good thing, and no one would ever for a second suggest going backwards. But even an accomplished student, a gifted artist, or a brilliant young law clerk is at a disadvantage if she never learned to write a thank-you note, understand a formal table setting, accept a compliment, make an apology, express sympathy, or respond to an invitation.

Learning these things will not cost you a cent, but knowing them and practicing them will without a shadow of a doubt pay enormous dividends, starting right now and lasting your lifetime.

The good news—for you and your parents—is that you don't have to add one more class to your overwhelming schedule. Within the pages of this book are small but very important lessons every young lady should know, whatever her dreams for her future may be.

Chapter 1

SAYING "PLEASE"

*W*hat was your first word? Your mother will probably tell you it was *Mama*. Your father will insist it was *Dada*. Your grandmother might even believe with all her heart that it was *Nana*. But *you* have no recollection. Chances are, though, that somewhere between Mama, Dada, and Nana, and before your first complete sentence, you learned the word *please*.

Your mother may have squatted down beside you, cookie in hand and said, "*Please*. I want a cookie, *please*," intending for you to repeat it back to her before rewarding you with the treat. Your dad may have sat down with you on the floor, ball in hand, and said, "*Please* play ball" before rolling it across the carpet to you. You also probably heard your parents use it with each other—"May I please have the paper when you're done with it?" "Will you please take the trash out?"— and saw the positive results.

Along with *mama, daddy, ball,* and *cookie, please* is one of the most important words you learn when you begin talking. It's hard to turn down someone who prefaces or ends a request with the word *please.* It doesn't matter if you are two years old and asking for a lollipop; eight years old and asking for a new backpack to replace the baby one from first grade; twelve years old and asking for money for a movie; fourteen and asking for a ride to the mall; or seventeen and asking a teacher to write a letter of recommendation for your college application. *Please* is a word that if you are smart—and considerate, which is just as important as being smart— you will use for the rest of your life.

You do

Say "please" consistently, to everyone, always. It doesn't matter if you're asking your brother to "pass the potatoes, please," or asking the busy clerk in the store to please wrap your purchase for your mother's birthday gift.

You don't

Treat your little brother, however annoying he may be, with any less consideration than you do a stranger. And vice versa.

Why

Because *please* really is a magic word that adds a layer of pleasantry to every request. The more you use it, the more natural it becomes to you.

A lady says the word *please* every time she makes a request, no matter how small it seems.

～

A lady answers, "Yes, please," if someone asks if she would like something. If not, she says, "No, thank you."

～

A lady knows "please" is just enough. Saying "pretty please" or "pleeeeeeeease" is unnecessary and can be annoying.

Chapter 2

SAYING "THANK YOU"

*H*as this ever happened to you? Your mother comes into your room while you are doing homework, lays your clean, folded laundry on your bed, stands by your desk for about ten seconds, then says, "You're welcome!" before she stomps out the door. Or your dad drops you off at your friend's house and as the car door is closing behind you, he shouts, "You're welcome!" This is not the time to roll your eyes; consider what you have *not* done that has irritated your mom or dad.

You might have "thank you" down pat when someone gives you something you've already asked for, but having good manners also means saying "thank you" after people do something nice when you haven't asked, or just out of the blue.

When your mom puts your clean laundry on your bed, when your dad gives you a ride, when your friend tells you how cute your outfit is, or her mom tells you after the soccer match what a great game you had, the response is as simple as "1,2, thank you."

You do

Say "thank you" anytime someone does something nice for you, no matter how well you know them.

You don't

Think you don't have to say "thank you" to your mom, your dad, or your big sister because they are family and don't count.

Why

Because family is where good manners begin, not where they end.

You do

Say "thank you" when a teacher compliments your drawing, or the piano teacher remarks kindly on your playing, even if you're not happy with your drawing or your performance.

You don't

Reply "it's ugly!" or "I was terrible!" even if you feel you could have done better.

Why

Because rejecting someone's kind comments on your accomplishment implies they have no taste, and that's insulting.

You do

Say "thank you" to the person who just made your strawberry-banana smoothie, handed you your change at the market, or gave you a program at the hockey game.

You don't

Assume that because people are "doing their jobs" they don't deserve to be thanked for that particular interaction with you.

Why

Because it makes people feel good to know their efforts are appreciated, and why wouldn't you want to make someone feel good?

A lady smiles and makes eye contact when she says "thank you."

A lady says "thank you" even when the person she is thanking is on the other end of the phone.

A lady says "thank you" even if no one else has—or *especially* if no one else has done so.

Chapter 3

SAYING "EXCUSE ME"

*W*hen it comes to the vocabulary of good manners, no phrase is more multifunctional or comes in handier than "excuse me."

You say "please" when asking for something and "thank you" when someone has done something for you or given you something nice. But "excuse me" has nearly as many uses as a Swiss Army pocketknife. It can be used as a request, as an attention getter, or as a type of apology when an apology isn't really necessary but not saying anything would be rude.

If you're walking down a crowded hall at school and happen to accidentally bump into someone, you say "excuse me."

If the only two remaining seats together at the movie theater are smack in the middle of the aisle, as you and your friend squeeze past each person, you should quietly say "excuse me." If you happen to step on the foot of someone who hasn't had the good sense to tuck it under his or her chair, you should add "I'm sorry."

If a group of people are chatting with one another and blocking a doorway you need to go through, you don't have to wait for them to move on; just say "excuse me" politely but loudly enough so they can hear you, and they'll let you right through.

If someone has spoken to you and you couldn't hear the entire sentence, you say "excuse me?" as a question, and they'll gladly repeat what they said.

In general, girls are far more careful than boys about belching at the table, but it happens, and when it does, there is no need to act as if it didn't. A simple "excuse me" is sufficient.

You do

Say "excuse me" if you have to walk through the middle of a line of people at the concession stand.

You don't

Scoot through when you see an opening as if no one will notice.

Why

People waiting in line can be very protective of their spots but will be happy to step back if they know your intention is not to butt in.

You do

Say "excuse me?" if you haven't heard what someone has said to you and would like them to repeat it.

You don't

Say "huh?"

Why

"Huh" sounds as if you are grunting, and young ladies don't grunt unless they are moving heavy objects or involved in an athletic endeavor.

You do

Say "excuse me" if you need to interrupt someone, even if it's your own mom on the computer or your dad reading a book.

You don't

Fidget, wave your arms around, or sigh dramatically.

Why

Because saying "excuse me" is a perfectly acceptable way to get someone's attention.

A lady always says "excuse me" to get someone's attention, not "hey" or "um."

～

A lady says "excuse me" when passing in front of someone's line of vision, whether that's in front of the lipstick display at the pharmacy or a painting in a museum.

Chapter 4

BEING INTRODUCED

*T*here's a reason that something is repeated over and over again, until it becomes one of those things that parents call "an old saying." It's because it has been tested by time and proven to be true. "The grass is always greener on the other side of the fence." "Don't count your chickens before they hatch." "The early bird gets the worm."

When your parents start a conversation with "There's an old saying . . . ," you should resist sighing loudly and instead listen to what they have to say, especially this: "You never get a second chance to make a first impression."

First impressions count, which is why the way you respond when being introduced to someone, especially an older someone, is very important.

Let's say your mother has dropped you off at your

father's office so he can take you to soccer practice. You are reading a magazine while you wait for him to pack up his briefcase. His boss walks into his office, and your father says, "Diana, this is my daughter Evelyn. Evelyn, this is Ms. Reid."

If you remain seated in your chair, barely look up over the top of the magazine, and mumble, "Hello" or even worse, "Hey," your father's boss will forever remember you as the rude young woman who didn't know the first thing about respect for older people.

When you are introduced to another person, the right thing to do is to look at the person and say, "It's nice to meet you Sam/Tressa/Mrs. Brooks/Mr. Tate/Reverend Stevens/Dr. Mayer." If the person you are being introduced to is your age, and it seems appropriate to shake hands, you can do so. If the person you are being introduced to is an adult, you wait for that person to extend their hand first, and if they do, offer a firm handshake, though not a tight grip.

If your father's boss walks into his office while you are reading a magazine, the first thing you do, even before your father gets one word out of his mouth, is close the magazine, set it on a table, and stand up. When your father says, "Diana, this is my daughter Evelyn. Evelyn, this is Ms. Reid," you make eye contact with Ms. Reid, smile, and say, "It's nice to meet you, Ms. Reid." If she extends her hand, shake it.

Five years down the road when you and your dad run into Ms. Reid in a restaurant or at a movie theater and he says to her, "Diana, do you remember my daughter Evelyn?" Ms. Reid will remember you as the very poised and polite young woman with impeccable manners whom she met in your father's office one afternoon. And that's certainly preferable to the alternative because one day you might want an internship or summer job at your father's company. You just never know.

You do

Repeat the person's name to whom you are being introduced.

You don't

Just say "hello" and think that covers it.

Why

Repeating a person's name back helps you remember their name for future reference, an invaluable asset.

You do

Stop what you are doing when you are being introduced.

You don't

Simply wave the hot dog you're eating at the ball game toward the person you're being introduced to.

Why

If someone thinks enough of you to introduce you to someone else, don't embarrass everyone—especially yourself—by acting as if you couldn't be bothered.

A lady smiles and makes eye contact with the person she is being introduced to.

~

A lady remembers that first impressions are lasting impressions.

~

If the person making introductions has somehow forgotten your name, a lady comes to the rescue by offering it herself. "Hello, I'm Mandy" is all that is needed to save the situation.

Chapter 5

MAKING INTRODUCTIONS

*I*f you've ever been invited to a birthday party for a girl you know from elementary school, but now you go to different middle schools and you don't really know any of her new friends, you were probably really anxious. You may have tried to get out of it by telling your mom, "But I don't know anybody." And your mom probably said, "You know Meaghan and it's her birthday and she invited you, so you're going. Besides, it's a chance to meet some new girls, and it's only two hours, and anybody can do anything for two hours."

That really didn't make you feel any better, and you were still a nervous wreck when you got there. But when Meaghan introduced you to her new friends and told them what a great soccer player you are and that her friend Carrie also played soccer, that gave you and Carrie something to talk about, and eventually you found out that Carrie also runs track in the spring and so does Laura. Before you knew it two hours had flown by, you had a great time, and you and Carrie had exchanged phone numbers.

Introductions are a way to help people feel included and as if they matter to you, so it is important to know how to properly make them.

If you are with one friend and run into another friend and you are all on your way somewhere else, it's enough to say, "Liza, this is Carrie. Carrie, this is Liza. We're going to a movie. Talk to you soon!" If you are all at the same party or event, you can add a bit more. "Liza, this is Meaghan. She and I went to Grassland Elementary together, but now she goes to Highlands Middle. Meaghan, Liza is on the soccer team with me at school."

If you are with your parents, you say, "Mom and Dad, this is Carrie. We met at Meaghan's party and she runs track for Highlands Middle." You do not need to add, "Carrie, these are my parents." That is pretty obvious.

If you are with your mother, and you run into your soccer coach at the post office, you say, "Mom, this is Coach Howe. She is my soccer coach." Your mom will probably already know that if she has been going to your games, but it never hurts to refresh someone's memory, especially when it comes to names.

You do

Include something personal about a friend you are introducing to your parents, like "Mom, this is Olga. She moved here from Germany last year."

You don't

Just say, "Mom, this is Olga."

Why

Because knowing a little something about your friend gives your parents an opening to get to know your friend a little better, which is reassuring for parents.

You do

Introduce a newcomer to a group of people she doesn't know, even if you don't know everyone's name in the group. You can simply say, "Everyone, this is Carrie. We went to elementary school together."

You don't

Say hello to the newcomer, then resume your conversation with your other friends.

Why

Not being introduced makes a person feel invisible and unimportant, and no one wants to make anyone feel that way.

A lady always introduces the younger person to the older person. "Grandma, this is Elizabeth." Not, "Elizabeth, this is my grandmother."

~

A lady can introduce herself to someone by saying her own name first. "Hello, I'm Jana Jones." Ideally, the other person will reply, "Hello, I'm Hannah Rogers."

Chapter 6

PAYING A COMPLIMENT

The expression "paying a compliment" is kind of funny because compliments are the gifts we give to others that don't cost a cent. They don't need to be sized, they don't need a box, and they don't have to be wrapped. But they are truly priceless.

A compliment only takes a few seconds to say, but it lingers for hours. When your mom is rushing out the door to work, and you tell her how great she looks in her new suit, she'll carry that with her all day long. When you tell your friend that the poem she wrote for English was so funny it made you laugh out loud, she'll remember that each time she reads it again. When you tell your grandmother that no one makes better biscuits than she does, she'll think of you each time she bakes up a batch.

Compliments are gifts that everyone loves getting and that never have to be taken back.

You do

Tell someone when you think she or he has done something really well, or when she looks really pretty, or when his jacket is really cool.

You don't

Keep those thoughts to yourself, even if you're shy or don't know the person that well. The opportunity will pass, and then you'll wish you had taken it.

Why

It is never wrong or incorrect to say something nice to someone.

You do

Pay compliments with sincerity and only when you mean it.

You don't

Say something nice just to have something to say.

Why

If you tell your friend every time you see her that she looks fantastic, she's going to stop believing you. Nobody, not even a supermodel, looks fantastic all the time.

PAYING A COMPLIMENT

A lady is not stingy with her compliments.

A lady does not exaggerate her compliments.

A lady is genuine in her compliments.

Chapter 7

ACCEPTING A COMPLIMENT

*Y*ou've probably told someone that you liked her dress, and she answered back, "It makes me look fat. I hate it." Or perhaps after a friend's piano recital you told him how much you enjoyed his playing, and he replied, "I was horrible! I totally messed up!" Or even one night at dinner you told your mom how good the chicken was, and she said, "You're kidding? I think I cooked it to death!"

Those responses weren't exactly what you were expecting, and they can leave you feeling kind of stupid—as if you were trying to insult your friend, or didn't know a thing about playing the piano, or had no taste at all.

As nice as compliments are to hear, it's amazing how many people—including grown-ups and otherwise really smart people—don't know how to receive them. But truthfully, it's so very simple. Two words will do. "Thank you." That's it. "Thank you."

You can add, "I appreciate you saying so" or "I'm glad you like it." But really, the most appropriate response to a compliment is "thank you."

You do

Say "thank you" when your friend tells you how cute your hair looks in a ponytail.

You don't

Say, "That's because I haven't washed it in four days!"

Why

No one needs to know your personal hygiene habits, and the appropriate response is "thank you."

You do

Say "thank you" when your teacher tells you how proud she is of your effort on your personal essay.

You don't

Say, "Really? I wrote it on the bus on the way to school this morning."

Why

Even if you did get away with such little effort on that assignment, do you really want to make your teacher feel foolish? The appropriate response is "thank you."

You do

Say "thank you" when your mother's friend tells you how much she likes your charcoal sketch in the school art show.

You don't

Say, "That piece? It's not very good."

Why

When someone compliments your accomplishments, it is rude to suggest that they have no idea what they're talking about. Even if in your heart you believe you could have done better, the appropriate response is "thank you."

⌒

A lady knows that accepting a compliment graciously is as important as giving a compliment sincerely, and she endeavors to do both.

Chapter 8

MAKING AN APOLOGY

*N*o one purposely sets out to hurt a friend's feelings, or let their father down. But it happens. As long as people do wrong, stupid, or hurtful things—even when they don't mean to—they will need to say "I'm sorry."

"I'm sorry" is a two-word phrase right up there with "thank you" and "excuse me" that makes the difference between thoughtful and thoughtless people, between kindness and rudeness, between civility and incivility. And you know which side of the line you want to be on.

Sometimes it seems hard to say "I'm sorry," but it's much harder to walk around with the burden of knowing you haven't tried to make amends for doing something harmful or hurtful to another person.

We all make mistakes and have accidents; we all do things, without thinking, that end up hurting other people; and we all have seen that our best intentions don't always result in doing the right thing.

That's when you say "I'm sorry." "I'm sorry I knocked into the table and broke your favorite piece of pottery." "I'm sorry I didn't include you when I went to the movies with Lacey and Anna Belle last weekend." "I'm sorry I forgot to take the dog out today and he made a mess on the rug."

And because it can be hard to say you're sorry, in the future you'll try harder not to make the same mistake again.

You do

Say "I'm sorry" without adding a "but."

You don't

Say, "I'm sorry I knocked into the table and broke your favorite piece of pottery, but you should have put it on a higher shelf if you liked it so much." You don't say, "I'm sorry I didn't include you with the others, but I was in a hurry." You don't say, "I'm sorry I forgot to let the dog out, but I wanted to watch the end of the show and he should have let me know he needed to go out."

Why

Adding an excuse to what you did or didn't do means you are not taking responsibility for your actions, and that makes your apology pretty worthless.

YOU DO

Say "I'm sorry and—" if you need to say more than "I'm sorry" to make the situation right. "I'm sorry I was careless and broke the bowl. Can I help buy a new one with my babysitting money?"

YOU DON'T

Assume that "I'm sorry" is always enough to make amends.

Why

Because as you get older you learn that sometimes you need to back up your words with action.

A lady doesn't delay her apology hoping the situation will just go away. It won't, and the sooner you say "I'm sorry," the sooner everyone feels better.

~

A lady doesn't expect to be rewarded for saying "I'm sorry" but is grateful when her apology is graciously accepted.

~

A lady doesn't assume an apology is the end of the situation, but she understands it's the first step toward making things right.

Chapter 9

ACCEPTING AN APOLOGY

*I*f your big brother teases you in front of his friends, it can really hurt your feelings. If your best friend borrows your favorite top and drips mustard all down the front, it's perfectly natural that you would get angry. If your mom promised to come to your volleyball game, and she got busy at work and completely forgot, you probably felt sad and mad.

If your brother or your friend or your mom doesn't come to you and say they're sorry for what they did or didn't do, you're just going to get more sad and more mad.

So when they do come to you and apologize— which, because they love you, they most likely will do—the right thing to do is accept their apology.

It can be hard, especially when you're still feeling

bad about what happened and want to be sure they know it. But chances are they do know, or they wouldn't be offering an apology. If your brother, your friend, or your mom says, "I know I hurt your feelings/ ruined your shirt/missed your game and I am really sorry," your response should be "I appreciate you saying so" or "I understand."

Your brother might do something nice to make up for being such a jerk, your friend will probably offer to replace your shirt, and your mom will do everything in her power not to miss another game.

Accepting someone's apology lets everyone start to feel better. It doesn't mean that what happened didn't matter. It means that being mature about it matters more.

You do

Say "that's okay" when someone apologizes to you.

You don't

Have to immediately give them a hug and act as if nothing happened.

Why

You have a right to feel hurt or angry when someone does something careless or hurtful. Sometimes it helps to take a little breather after the apology is offered and accepted.

You do

Say "I appreciate your apology" when someone apologizes to you.

You don't

Say, "I appreciate your apology . . . but you are really a jerk/you should have been more careful/you really made me feel terrible . . . don't do it again."

Why

Replying to an apology with a qualifier is not really accepting an apology.

You do

Forgive someone when they have done something careless or hurtful to you.

You don't

Forget it if they do the same thing over and over.

Why

Being a lady doesn't mean allowing people to take advantage of you and your good nature. If the same thing happens more than once, it's time to sit down and talk it over.

A lady accepts an apology
without conditions.

~

A lady does not keep reminding her
brother, her friend, or her mother of
their transgression once the apology
is accepted.

~

A lady knows how to forgive
and in time, forget.

~

A lady does not hold a grudge.

Chapter 10

ASKING PERMISSION

*A*s long as there have been children eager to grow up—which there always have been— at some point in their lives, they have been frustrated at being denied permission to do something, and in frustration they have said, "I can't wait until I grow up and I can do whatever I want." That's not ever going to happen.

When you were really little, you used to have to ask someone older or bigger than you for almost everything because you weren't big enough to do it yourself. You couldn't reach the cookie jar or pour a glass of milk. You couldn't just toddle across the street by yourself to see your friend or climb up onto the chair and turn the family computer on to play a game.

Once you get older and bigger, you don't need to ask for as much help, but in many cases you do need to ask permission. Your father doesn't just walk over to the neighbor's garage and take his hedge clippers; he asks permission to borrow them. Your grandmother doesn't just jump in the car to take off for a weekend with "the girls" in New Orleans. (Yes, grandmothers call their girlfriends "the girls" long after they've aged out of girlhood. You will too.) She checks first with your grandfather to see if it's okay or if he has other plans.

Asking permission is something you do from a very young age—like asking your kindergarten teacher for permission to take a puzzle off the shelf— to a very old age. No matter how old you are, asking for permission is something you never outgrow.

You do

Ask permission to use your mom's laptop, borrow your friend's French-English dictionary, ride your bike to the ballpark, or stay out an hour past your curfew.

You don't

Assume that it's okay to do any of those things because you're not nine years old anymore, or because you've done them before.

Why

Each time you use something that belongs to someone else or do something out of the ordinary, you ask permission.

You do

Offer an explanation of why you need to use your mom's laptop or stay out an hour past your curfew.

You don't

Ask for permission without being prepared for a follow-up question and response.

Why

Your mom might need to use her laptop herself, but if you tell her there's a program you need on the laptop for a paper you're writing and you promise to give it back in one hour, she'll probably say yes.

You do

Accept no as a final answer when it's clear that's what the answer is going to be.

You don't

Whine, cry, stomp your foot, and accuse your parents of always saying no, being totally unfair, and hating you.

Why

Accepting no for an answer with maturity will impress your parents so much that they are far more likely to say yes the next time. If you sense yourself getting upset, you might want to go to your room to cool down. If it helps, you can yell into your pillow.

A lady never uses or borrows something that belongs to someone else without asking permission. No exceptions.

～

A lady doesn't change the radio station in the car her mom is driving without asking permission.

～

A lady doesn't stay out past curfew or go to a different place than she told her parents she was going without asking permission first.

Chapter 11

ASKING FOR A FAVOR

There's a fine line between asking for an occasional favor, and asking someone to do something inappropriate or beyond the call of friendship.

If you've had to stay home sick, asking your classmate who carpools with you to pick up your school assignments and drop them by your house is a favor anyone would be happy to do. Asking a friend for some help with a question you don't understand is also a favor. Asking a friend if you can copy their homework because you've missed a few days of school and don't understand the assignment is crossing the line and putting your friend in a very uncomfortable position.

Asking your little brother to cover your chore of walking the dog one afternoon after school because you have a huge paper due the next day is a favor. Asking your little brother to walk the dog every day for a week is taking advantage of your status in the birth order and is guaranteed to make him mad enough to tell your parents.

Asking your teammates if it's okay to leave right after practice and not help collect and put away the equipment because your big sister is picking you up and you're going out for dinner is a favor. Skipping out on your duties as a member of a team on a regular basis makes you a bad teammate, and is certain to foster bad feelings.

Knowing the difference now between asking for a favor and taking advantage of someone's good nature will be even more important as you get older and need bigger favors. When you go to the mountains for a week with your family and you ask your friend to come to your house every day to feed your cat, the right thing to do is bring your friend a small token of appreciation—a cute souvenir, a box of candy, a bar of soap. In the not too distant future, when you're going to college six hours away, you might need a ride home for fall break. The right thing to do is offer to fill the driver's car with gas.

A favor is an act of kindness someone does for you beyond what is due; a lady doesn't take advantage or fail to express her appreciation.

You do

Ask for a favor only when you're in a pinch and really need it.

You don't

Ask for favors over and over from the same person.

Why

The person you keep asking will understandably begin to avoid you.

You do

Acknowledge the favor you have received.

You don't

Take advantage of a person's kindness or inability to say no to you.

Why

Word travels among friends and you don't want to get a reputation as a user.

A lady says "thank you" when her brother agrees to cover dog-walking duty that day, and again after he does it.

⤔

A lady offers to reciprocate a favor, telling her brother, for example, that if he walks the dog for her, she will cover one of his chores.

⤔

A lady gets someone who does a big favor for her a small token of appreciation.

Chapter 12

BORROWING CLOTHES

$\mathcal{G}$irls borrow clothes from one another as casually and naturally as boys poke each other in the ribs and see who can eat the most pizza. But there is some basic protocol to be aware of when borrowing a friend's clothes.

Borrowing clothes can be preplanned. If you know that Brittney has an adorable baby-blue sweater that will go perfectly with your brown jeans, you might call or text her and ask if you can borrow her adorable baby-blue sweater to wear to the movie on Friday night.

Or borrowing clothes can be an act comparable to spontaneous combustion when two or more girls gather at one house to get ready to go out—"out" being anything from walking four blocks down the street to the park where the boys' soccer team practices or to a kick-off-the-seventh-grade party in the school gym.

Girls arrive at the staging house carrying tote bags stuffed with potential outfits to audition for the other girls. The hostess's closet is raided, and by the time the group leaves the house, no one is wearing anything—except underwear—that belongs to them.

You do

Ask before borrowing an article of clothing, pair of boots, or piece of jewelry from a friend, a sister, or your mom.

You don't

Take something thinking they won't mind or that you'll get it back before they notice.

Why

Borrowing something without asking is almost like stealing and you would never do that. Besides, you are bound to run into the person you "borrowed" the plaid skirt from while you are wearing it.

You do

Understand the boundaries for what is acceptable to borrow.

You don't

Borrow underwear, makeup, hairbrushes, or anything with the tags still on it.

Why

Borrowing underwear is far too intimate, even for sisters. Sharing makeup or hairbrushes may result in sharing far more than you bargained for. The first person to wear a new article of clothing should always be the person who owns it.

You do

Return the item of clothing cleaned, wrinkle-free, folded, or on a hanger.

You don't

Return a dirty shirt, a knotted necklace, or mud-spattered shoes.

Why

Being a responsible borrower is as important as being a courteous houseguest. You are a temporary caretaker of someone else's property.

You do

Return what you borrowed in a timely fashion.

You don't

Wait until the person you borrowed something from has to come and retrieve it.

Why

Borrowing is a temporary lease, not a permanent trade or purchase.

⁓

A lady does not borrow something that she knows is too small for her.

⁓

A lady launders or dry-cleans clothing that she borrows before returning it.

⁓

A lady replaces something she borrows with the identical item if she stains, tears, or otherwise makes the item unwearable. If that is not possible, she offers to reimburse her friend with cash for the ruined item.

Chapter 13

TALKING AND LISTENING TO ADULTS

*Y*ou might think you have this one covered since
you've been talking and listening to your parents
your whole life.

That is only partially correct.

As you mature, your level of interaction with
others should mature as well. The circle of people you
interact with will also grow, from your parents and
grandparents to your teachers, coaches, counselors,
employers, parents of friends, and random grown-
ups you will encounter throughout the course of your
adolescence.

While the tone of conversations you have with

family members will be more casual than the tone of conversations you have with your teacher or your advisor or the librarian, all require the same thing: your full attention.

This means that when your mother comes into your room to talk to you about the slumber party you're planning, you stop texting. If you're in the middle of sending a text, you let your mother know that—"I'll just tell Molly I'll get back to her"—and then you put the phone away.

If your teacher wants to talk to you about your assignment, you make eye contact and let her know by your responses that you are absorbing what she is saying.

If you need help from the librarian, you take out your earbuds before you ask where you might find a book.

When you are making a purchase at the convenience store, you stop talking to your friend on your cell phone and engage with the cashier.

As you get older, you will be expected to initiate conversation with grown-ups, and you can practice with your parents and grandparents. It's not hard. Just ask a question. "How was your day at work, Mom?" "What are you reading, Grandpa?" "Who do you think will win the Super Bowl, Dad?" And then, listen to their answer.

Showing interest in other people's lives is one of the most courteous things you can do, and an important milestone on your way to maturity.

You do

Stop texting on your phone, typing on the computer, or watching television when an adult wants to speak with you.

You don't

Make a show of being irritated at the interruption, or act as if you are impatient to get back to what you were doing.

Why

There are distractions all around us, but grown-ups should not have to vie with a friend you saw an hour ago at school or with reruns of *Gilmore Girls* for five minutes of your time. It is hurtful to feel that you are not worthy of someone's undivided attention.

You do

Politely ask your mom if her question can wait two more minutes for the outcome of the tie-breaking tennis match, or until you finish your train of thought on the paper you're writing.

You don't

Put your hand up in front of her face, or wave her away like an annoying fly.

Why

Either of those things is guaranteed to provoke an angry response, which will not get you the two minutes you've requested.

You do

Initiate conversations with the grown-ups in your life.

You don't

Spend all your time "conversing" on the computer with friends and strangers or secluded in your bedroom.

Why

As you're getting older, so are your parents and grandparents, and it's important to make the most of the time we have with the people we love.

A lady makes eye contact and is engaged with the person she is conversing with.

A lady knows that asking people questions about themselves is the surest way to be considered a good conversationalist.

A lady keeps up with current events and popular culture, at least enough to learn the art of small talk.

Chapter 14

BEING A DINNER GUEST

*I*t may be as casual as your friend's mom suggesting you stay for supper after you finish studying together, or you may receive a formal invitation to a celebratory dinner of some type. Doing the right thing is usually a matter of following the lead of your hostess, though it helps to know some basic rules of being a guest at the dinner table. Here are some guidelines.

- Do not sit at the table before anyone else or after everyone else, but at the same time as most of the other guests.
- Unless your hostess tells everyone to start without her, do not begin eating before the hostess is also seated at the table and lifts her fork.

- If you are serving yourself from a buffet, do not heap your plate with food as if you are storing up for the winter; instead take only as much as you know you can eat at that sitting.
- Do not put something on your plate, then change your mind and put it back on the platter or in the bowl. Once it is on your plate, it is yours.
- Never take anything from a buffet with your hand when a serving piece is provided.
- If serving dishes are being passed around the table family style, the proper direction is counterclockwise, to the right. But if everyone is passing clockwise to the left, do as they do.
- Take just one piece of bread from the basket, and pass it along. If you are asked to pass the breadbasket that is sitting in front of you, do not snatch a roll before sending the basket on its way.
- Do not reach across others to get something you need; ask for it to be passed to you. If someone asks you for the salt, pass the salt and pepper shakers together, so one doesn't get separated from the other. Do not pass across the table, but to the right until the item gets to the person who requested it.

Though guests at a table should participate in the conversation as they are able, never chew with your mouth open or talk with your mouth full. If you feel a sneeze or cough coming on, turn your head away from the table and cover your mouth.

Hairbrushes, makeup, and cell phones have no place at the table. Ever.

You do

Compliment the food.

You don't

Go on and on about how the chicken casserole is the best chicken casserole you have ever tasted in your whole life and how it is so much better than your mother's.

Why

Overflattering can be perceived as insincere, and comparing your mother's cooking to anyone else's in derogatory terms is a breach of family protocol.

You do

Ask if anyone else would like the last piece of chicken or last roll before you claim it.

You don't

Take the last of anything without checking with the rest of the table.

Why

It is highly unlikely that anyone else will thwart your wish for another roll, but they should be given the option. If someone else also had their eye on the last piece of bread, they should suggest sharing it.

YOU DO

Say "excuse me" if you need to get up from the table to use the restroom.

YOU DON'T

Abruptly jump up and run off, even if the need is urgent.

Why

It only takes one second to say "excuse me" and you don't have to explain why.

YOU DO

Offer to help clear the table, serve dessert, or clean up after dinner.

YOU DON'T

Insist when the host or hostess declines.

Why

Your hostess will certainly appreciate your thoughtfulness in asking, but no means no. She may not want you getting in her way or may prefer to clean up after her guests depart.

～

A lady arrives on time for a meal, leaves her cell phone on vibrate in another room, and keeps her elbows off the table.

～

If it is her host family's custom to say a blessing before a meal, a lady follows their lead.

～

A lady always thanks the host family for including her before she departs.

Chapter 15

THE NAPKIN

*I*f you have spent your entire life so far eating at the kitchen table with your family; if even holiday and birthday dinners are extremely casual affairs with disposable plates and plastic cutlery; and if the only places you have eaten out are restaurants where you order, pay for, and receive your food from a counter, then you are probably familiar with paper napkins.

Soon enough, though, you will be a guest at a dinner with cloth napkins. The good news is that proper usage of cloth napkins is pretty much the same as with paper napkins. The bad news is that if you don't know basic, proper napkin usage, that will be much more noticeable on occasions involving cloth napkins. Again, the good news is that napkin rules are pretty simple.

As soon as you are seated, take the napkin from

beside your plate, unfold it, and place it across your lap.

Keep it in your lap unless you need to wipe your fingers or mouth—not your entire face. (It's a napkin, not a washcloth.)

When you are finished eating, place your napkin back on the table beside your plate, loosely folded and not wadded up in a ball.

You do

Unfold your napkin and lay it in your lap.

You don't

Unfurl your napkin and give it a big shake.

Why

A napkin is not a flag, and you don't want to slap someone as a result of your theatrics.

You do

Use your napkin to wipe your fingers as needed, particularly if the menu includes messy items like chicken wings or corn on the cob.

You don't

Lick your fingers.

Why

    Licking one's fingers is something only done in solitude, without witnesses. You are at a civilized table, not stranded on a desert island.

You do

Use your napkin to cover your mouth if you start coughing or have to sneeze.

You don't

Blow your nose on your napkin.

Why

    Do you really want to use a germ-covered napkin to blot your lips? If you need to blow your nose, excuse yourself from the table and find a tissue.

A lady who is old enough to wear lipstick blots her lips on a tissue before coming to the table so she doesn't leave stains on her napkin or marks on her drinking glass.

~

A lady leaves her loosely folded napkin on her seat if she has to get up from the table for any reason before the meal is over.

~

If a lady's napkin falls to the floor, she quickly picks it up and puts it back on her lap.

~

A lady puts her napkin on the table beside her plate—not on it—when she is finished eating, as a signal that her plate may be cleared.

Chapter 16

THE PLACE SETTING

*R*emember the first time you opened your Spanish textbook and nothing made sense to you? There were words on the page made of letters you knew, but you had no idea what they meant or how to say them.

You will probably feel the same way the first time you sit down to a formal dinner, one with lots of utensils and glasses and different plates. They all look familiar, but how does it work?

You might get really nervous about doing the wrong thing, using the wrong fork, or drinking out of someone else's glass. It's actually quite logical and simpler than you might guess.

Square the area around your plate—to the left, right, and immediately above—as your "property." Solids—like the small plate for your bread—are to the left, and liquids—like your drinking glass—are to the right. One easy way to remember is to imagine a small *b* to the left and a small *d* to the right; *b* is for bread, *d* is for drink.

As for utensils, you just work your way in, course by course. Forks are always placed to the left of the plate, and knives and spoons to the right of the plate. If there is a fork and spoon placed horizontally at the top of your plate, those are intended for dessert and you don't need to think about them until your pie or cake is delivered to you.

A small butter knife may be laid across the bread plate. That knife is only to be used for buttering your bread. It is not to be used for taking butter off the butter plate. There will be a separate knife for that, and you will use it to put some butter on your bread plate, but not on your bread.

Once you have used a utensil, you do not lay it on the table again. If you are still eating, you can prop the tines of the fork or the end of the knife on the edge of your plate.

The meal might begin with a salad; the salad fork is smaller than the dinner fork and will be on the outside to the left of the plate. That is the one you begin with. If you must use a knife to cut your salad, rest the knife on the salad plate until it is cleared, then rest it on your bread plate until your main course is served. If there is no bread plate, simply prop it on the spoon.

If the meal starts with soup, there will be a larger soupspoon outside the teaspoon on the right of your plate.

When the main course is served, you will have the main fork and your knife left to use. When you are not using your knife, prop or rest it on the plate.

When you are finished with your meal, place your knife and fork—tines down and pointed to the upper left corner—side by side, diagonally across your plate.

YOU DO

Use the water glass to the right of your plate.

YOU DON'T

Drink from more than one water glass if you have gotten mixed up.

Why

Everyone has made this mistake, especially people who are left-handed, and it is no big deal. Tell the person to your left you have used their glass and give them the one you have not used.

YOU DO

Pace your eating to the rest of the table.

You don't

Gobble your food—even if you are famished—or eat at a snail's pace.

Why

You do not want to sit and watch everyone else eat if your plate is emptied well before theirs; neither does everyone else want to wait for you to finish so they can get their cherry pie.

You do

Put your utensils on your plate if you must pause to pass the breadbasket or wipe your mouth.

You don't

Lay dirty utensils on the table.

Why

You don't want to leave grease stains or tomato sauce on the tablecloth.

A lady does not push food onto her fork with her finger, but uses a piece of bread or the edge of her knife.

⌒

If a lady drops a utensil on the floor, she does not pick it up and wipe it on her napkin, but asks for a replacement.

⌒

A lady does not butter an entire roll or slice of bread at one time, but only the piece she is about to put into her mouth.

Chapter 17

FOOD ALLERGIES
AND DISLIKES

*E*veryone has some kind of food they don't like,
kids especially. When you were really little,
your mom probably worried you'd never eat anything
but Cheerios, chicken fingers, macaroni and cheese,
French fries, pizza, and grilled cheese sandwiches for
the rest of your life.

As you get older, your taste and taste buds mature
as well, but there will always be those one or two
things that you just can't abide, that might even make
you sick just thinking about them. Maybe it's beets
or Brussels sprouts or peas or peanut butter or tuna.
Maybe it's all of those things.

When you're eating at home, your mom or dad,
or whoever does the cooking for your family, already
knows that about you, and their feelings won't be hurt

if you don't eat those things. When you're a guest in someone's home or at a special dinner and lima beans are being passed around the table, it's a little trickier, but it's still manageable.

Food allergies are much more serious and your parents have probably taught you never to eat foods you are allergic to, no matter how delicious or harmless they look. If strawberries make you break out in a rash all over your body, shellfish make you vomit, or peanuts send you into shock, you need to share that with your host or hostess. No one wants to be responsible for making someone sick.

You do

Just pass along without comment a dish of something you know you hate.

You don't

Make a face and say, "I think beets are so gross! How can you eat those things?"

Why

Making faces and blurting disparaging comments about food that is being served to you is a good way to ensure you won't be invited back.

You do

Let a friend who asks you to dinner know in advance

if you have severe food allergies so she can share that with the cook.

You don't

Wait until everyone is sitting at the table for a shrimp boil, sigh loudly, and tell them the only thing you can eat is the bread.

Why

It's awkward for everyone else at the table if one person isn't eating. Letting your host or hostess know in advance allows them to prepare something that won't send you to the hospital.

You do

Take a little bit of something you've never tried.

You don't

Spit something out of your mouth if it turns out you hate it, hide the rest of it under a piece of bread, or drop it in your napkin.

Why

When you take just a little bit of an unfamiliar food, you might discover something you really love, and asking for more will please the cook. If you find you don't like it, it's not rude to leave just that small bit on your plate.

Food Allergies and Dislikes

A lady lets her host or hostess know in advance if her religious beliefs prevent her from eating a particular food, or she is a vegetarian or vegan.

～

A lady doesn't need to say how much she hates lima beans if they are offered to her; she simply says, "No, thank you. But I'd love some more salad!"

～

A lady doesn't point out how fattening something is, even if it is very fattening.

Chapter 18

DINING IN A RESTAURANT

*G*oing out to eat in a restaurant is similar to being
a guest in someone's house, except that you
don't know the people who are serving you, and you
probably won't ever see them again. That doesn't mean
you shouldn't follow the same rules and be just as
courteous as you would be in your friend's house or at
your grandmother's.

Different restaurants have different levels of
formality, from bare tables and plastic forks to thick
linen tablecloths and real silver. But there will always
be a napkin to put on your lap and there will always be
cutlery to use properly; your water glass will always be
to your right and your bread plate to your left.

The biggest difference between being a guest in
a home and a patron in a restaurant is that in a home,

everyone eats whatever the host has prepared. In a restaurant, you may choose—within reason—what you want to eat.

When you were little and couldn't read, a grown-up at the table ordered for you. Later, the server may have handed you a special children's menu that included your favorites like spaghetti, hot dogs, and chicken fingers. Almost always, these meals included a drink and a dessert, and they were all the same price. Once you decided between the cheeseburger and the pizza, you didn't have to give it another thought.

Now that you've aged out of the cute placemats, crayons, and kiddie meals, you'll be given a real menu. You might see lots of items with ingredients you've never heard of; that can be intimidating, even for grown-up experienced diners.

But no one is going to let you go hungry; you can always ask an adult at the table or the server to tell you more about the dish.

You do

Aim for the middle of the price range if you are dining out as a guest.

You don't

Order the most expensive item or the least expensive item on the menu, unless the least expensive item is your favorite thing.

Why

Your host is trusting you to make good decisions, and ordering a $50 steak when she orders the $25 salmon is not a good decision. On the other hand, ordering something you don't like just because it is the cheapest thing on the menu is wasteful if you don't eat it.

You do

Ask your server to explain a dish you are not familiar with.

You don't

Order "steak tartare with farm egg yolk" because you recognize the words *steak* and *egg*—especially when your server raises an eyebrow and says, "Are you sure?"

Why

You will probably be quite shocked when a plate of raw ground beef topped by a raw egg is set before you. Not understanding what you are ordering can have very unpleasant results.

You do

Speak up—politely and discreetly—to whichever grown-up at the table is the host, if your meal is unsatisfactory.

You don't

Suffer through an ice-cold steak or a soup so oversalted your tongue curls.

Why

Restaurants count on satisfied customers to remain in business. If you don't speak up at the restaurant, they don't have a chance to correct their error. On the other hand, you don't need to throw a fit about it or let an entire plate of food go to waste.

A lady waits until everyone has received their meal before she begins eating.

~

A lady may politely ask if her salad can be made without onions, or if she might have Swiss cheese rather than cheddar on her cheeseburger.

~

A lady knows to tip at least 15 percent if she is eating with friends and everyone is responsible for their own check.

~

A lady treats all restaurant staff—from the manager to the busboys—with respect.

Chapter 19

PUBLIC STAIRCASES AND HALLWAYS

*I*magine what roads and highways would look like if everyone just drove wherever they wanted. Or what chaos would ensue if there were no designated runways for planes or designated turns for takeoffs and landings.

Traffic in public hallways, on staircases and escalators, and through doors doesn't have the same potential for disaster as on interstates and in airports, but there are certain guidelines to follow to keep things flowing in an orderly fashion.

Most of these rules are just common sense and follow the same rules of real roads, but they can be forgotten when we're in a hurry.

You do

Stay to the right while walking in a hall and ascending or descending a staircase.

You don't

Walk on the left, walk in the middle, or drift from side to side.

Why

In America, we drive on the right and we walk the same way. In two-way traffic, keeping everyone to their right avoids bumps and collisions of the vehicular and pedestrian variety.

You do

Stay to the right side of an ascending or descending escalator.

You don't

Anchor yourself in the middle.

Why

Some people are in a hurry and prefer to walk rather than ride escalators; when they pass riders, they need to have access to the left side of the moving staircase.

You do

Watch where you are going and pay attention to your surroundings and the people around you in public places.

You don't

Walk and text, make sudden stops in hallways or midway up a staircase, or pause at the top or bottom of an escalator.

Why

You will most certainly be rear-ended and could hurt yourself and others, perhaps causing a dangerous pile up.

A lady passes slower walkers to their left, and says "excuse me" as she does so, doing her best not to startle the other walker.

Ladies do not walk more than two abreast in a hallway, on a walking path, or on a staircase. If the hallway is narrow, with oncoming traffic, ladies walk in single file until lanes are clear.

~

A lady steps to the rear or side of an elevator when other passengers enter. If it is quite crowded and she is closest to the panel, she asks "which floor?" and pushes the appropriate button. If someone is having trouble getting out, she pushes the button that holds the door open.

~

Ladies hold a door for older people, people with packages, and people pushing strollers. If someone holds a door for her, she always says "thank you."

Chapter 20

CHOOSING AND GIVING A GIFT

When you were a little girl, you probably made something in art class for special occasions like Christmas, Hanukkah, and Mother's Day. Those pinecones covered in glue and glitter, little handprints in a plaster of Paris plate, and picture frames made of popsicle sticks will be treasured long after you have moved along to choosing store-bought gifts for friends and family.

The reason they mean so much is because they took time and effort, a rule of thumb for gift giving we should never outgrow.

It doesn't matter if you don't have much money to spend. With a little time and effort, you can find just the right gift.

You do

Take note of people's favorite colors, music, movies, books, and hobbies.

You don't

Pick something because you like it.

Why

You give someone a gift you are fairly certain they will enjoy. You don't give a friend who loves the color red a pink cardigan because that's *your* favorite color. Pink might be in the red family, but the two colors don't really get along, and she will probably never wear the sweater.

You do

Plan ahead and keep track of birthdays on a dry-erase board or calendar in your bedroom, or on your computer or phone.

You don't

Wait until the last minute to look for your mother's Christmas present or a gift for your friend's birthday.

Why

Choosing just the right gift should be fun, but if you put it off until the last minute, you'll get stressed. And what's worse, it becomes a chore, which will likely result in your choosing a present that fairly shouts "She waited until the last minute!" You don't have to wait until department stores are playing "Deck the Halls" to shop for Christmas. If you see a pair of earrings in September you know your mother will love, buy them and hide them away. (Just don't forget where you put them.) If you know your friend is going on a cruise with her family for winter break, monogrammed luggage tags for her October birthday show you've thought ahead.

You do

Take the time to wrap your gift nicely or put it in a fun gift bag.

You don't

Hand it to the recipient in the bag from the store where it was purchased or in the box it was mailed in.

Why

Which present would you look forward to opening more? The one in the wrinkled-up brown paper bag or the one in the polka-dot shiny paper with a big satin bow? Don't be the person who brings the wrinkled-up brown paper bag. If you don't have a knack for wrapping, use a gift bag, colorful tissue, and some pretty ribbon.

A lady always removes the price tag and puts a gift receipt with the item if the store offers one, in case the item has to be exchanged for any reason.

A lady includes a card or tag with her name on packages or in gift bags.

A lady doesn't say, "If you don't like it, you can take it back" to the recipient as he or she is opening their gift. It is awkward and uncomfortable.

Chapter 21

ACCEPTING A GIFT

What's so hard about accepting a gift? You just open it up and say "thank you." Sooner rather than later, your mom will hand you a pile of note cards and a pen and tell you not to leave the house until you write your thank-you notes.

Other than saying "thank you," there aren't really rules about accepting gifts, but there are niceties we observe—even when your great-aunt Hazel gives you a sweater that is clearly three sizes too big and smells suspiciously like Aunt Hazel. Or your grandmother gives you this book, when you were hoping for a gift card to Sephora.

No matter what the gift is, the point is that someone has taken the time and effort to choose it just for you, wrapped it, and given it to you with the natural expectation that the gesture will be appreciated.

You do

Say "thank you" as soon as you open the gift.

You don't

Say, "Oh, I already have this book" or "This really isn't my color."

Why

Even if you do have the book or fuchsia does make you look ill, "thank you" is the only appropriate response for any and every gift you receive. You don't have to lie and say, "Oh, I love fuchsia!" But you do say, "Thank you for the pretty sweater, Aunt Hazel."

You do

Take time to acknowledge every gift you open when there are many gifts to be opened—at your birthday party, for example.

You don't

Tear through packages as if you're trying to beat the clock.

Why

When you are opening your gifts at a birthday party, it is part of the fun for your guests to see and admire what everyone else has brought. Opening gifts at a more leisurely pace also allows you to keep the cards with the gifts, which will be important later when you sit down to write thank-you notes.

You do

Say something nice about each gift you receive.

You don't

Go on and on about one particular gift and barely acknowledge the others.

Why

Yes, the Tiffany key chain may be something one of your friends, with the means to afford it, knows you have coveted for months. But effusive gushing over the key chain will make it appear you like that gift more than any of the others you have received. Even if you do, you can save your rave for the thank-you note you write to your generous friend.

A lady says "thank you" for every gift, the ones she loves and the ones she doesn't.

∿

A lady never points out to the giver that she already has the gift she just opened.

∿

A lady can think of something nice to say about every gift she receives. "Thank you for the *Figaro* CD, Uncle Harold. It will be my first opera!"

∿

A lady does not announce the amount of a check her grandmother has enclosed in her birthday card. She simply says, "Thank you, Nana" and puts the check back in the card.

Chapter 22

WRITING A THANK-YOU NOTE

*K*nowing when to write a thank-you note is easy: you write a thank-you note whenever someone does something really nice for you or gives you a gift.

Knowing how to write a thank-you note is a little bit harder, but once you've got the hang of it, you'll want to make a habit of it. Expressing your appreciation for something in a brief but sincere note isn't something you outgrow. In fact, it's a skill and a courtesy that will become even more important as you get older and need to acknowledge graduation gifts, job interviews, and wedding presents.

A well-written personal note always impresses people—whether that person is your grandmother, your best friend's parents, or the person you hope to call your boss. It especially stands out when the habits of more casual correspondence have made thank-you notes seem exceptional. Being exceptional is always a good thing.

You do

Write a thank-you note for a gift you've received.

You don't

Think that saying "thank you" in person when you receive the gift is enough or that texting "thx!" will take care of it.

Why

    If someone has taken the time and effort to choose and purchase a gift for you, the most meaningful way to respond is to express your appreciation in writing.

You do

Write your thank-you notes as promptly as possible.

You don't

Think that because you have procrastinated for a month or more after your birthday, there's no sense in sending a note so late.

Why

Sooner is better than later, but late is better than never. If a month has gone past since you received the watch from your grandmother, you might start with a quick apology for your tardiness, and even make a little joke about how you hope it makes you more timely. You do not say, "I've been so busy, I didn't have time." You don't need to offer an excuse, just an apology.

YOU DO

Write your friend's parents a thank-you note for taking you to the beach with them for spring break.

YOU DON'T

Write your friend's mother a thank-you note for giving you a ride home from the movie.

Why

Some things—like a ride home or asking you to stay for pizza with the family—are simply considerations that people do for others in the course of daily life. Bringing you along for a vacation, taking you as their guest to a really nice restaurant, or inviting you to use one of the family's football season tickets are all special, and should be acknowledged as such.

You do

Say something personal and specific in your thank-you note.

You don't

Write something that sounds like a form letter for which you have filled in the blanks.

Why

People want to know that their gift or gesture has made an impression on you in some way. Writing "Dear Aunt Molly, Thank you for the gift you sent me. Sincerely, Anna Belle" is impersonal and vague.

A lady handwrites a thank-you note on a note card or stationery, not on a piece of paper torn out of a notebook.

A lady uses her best handwriting,
even if that means printing.
An illegible note can lead to
miscommunication or even a
headache for the person attempting
to read it.

Here are a couple of examples you can use as guidelines.

Dear Grandma,

I love the sweater you made me for Christmas! Whenever I wear something you knitted, I get so many compliments on it, and I know this sweater will be admired too. Thank you so much for all the work you put into it. I will think of you every time I wear it.

Love,
Anna Belle

Dear Mr. and Mrs. Green,

I had the best time at the beach with your family during spring break. I love looking at all the photos Susan and I took and seeing how much fun we had. Thank you so much for including me and making me feel so welcome. I will always remember it.

Sincerely,
Anna Belle Carter

Dear Uncle Bob,

Thank you so much for the generous check you sent for my birthday. I am saving up to buy a laptop computer and your check will go toward that goal. It was very thoughtful of you to remember my day. I hope to see you soon.

Love,
Anna Belle

Chapter 23

EXPRESSING SYMPATHY

*R*emember how when you were little, everything seemed so easy? If you wanted to play soccer, your mom or dad just signed you up for the team that all your friends were on, and everybody played, even if you never once scored a goal. All the parents sat on the sideline cheering, and after the game you had juice and snacks. When the season was over, at a pizza party every member of the team got a trophy for something.

When you were in first grade, everyone got a medal or a ribbon during field day; and in third grade everyone got to have their drawing displayed in the mall for the art show.

As you get older, the standards to which people are held as athletes, artists, musicians, and students get tougher. There will be disappointments for you and your friends.

It can be hard to know what to say when your friend doesn't make the volleyball team, or the cheerleading squad, or the string quartet, or the juried art show, or the Honor Society because of one stupid test.

It's even more difficult to know what to say when truly sad things happen. Like a pet dying, or even worse, a grandparent or other close relative. These things will happen as we get older. Grown-ups get just as nervous about what to say at such sad times; they've just had more practice.

You do

Say, "I'm sorry that you didn't make the volleyball team" or "I'm sorry you didn't win the election for Student Council president."

You don't

Criticize the people who did make the team or person who was voted president.

Why

Saying bad things about other people won't do anything to make your friend feel better. In fact, it might make her feel worse. Acknowledge your friend's disappointment, listen to what she has to say, then move on. Losing an election for freshman class president is not the end of the world.

You do

Say, "I'm so sorry that your dog Millie died. She was so cute and funny."

You don't

Say, "I'm sorry to hear that Millie died. When are you going to get another dog?"

Why

As anyone who has ever had and loved a dog or cat or horse or even a ferret knows, pets are unique and irreplaceable. Someday your friend might get another dog, but she needs time to mourn the one she has lost.

You do

Say, "I am sorry to hear that your grandmother died. I know you were very close."

You don't

Say, "I'm sorry to hear that your grandmother died. I know just how you feel."

Why

Every relationship is unique, and so is every loss. Even if your grandmother passed away recently, you really don't know just how your friend feels about her grandmother's death. If you knew your friend's grandmother and want to say something nice about her, such as "Your grandmother had the most beautiful smile" or "Your grandmother made the best chocolate cake ever," that would be a thoughtful memory for your friend to hear.

You do

Take the time to listen if your friend wants to talk about her loss.

You don't

Change the subject or suddenly remember somewhere else you have to be.

Why

People say, "I wish there was something I could do." Just being there and listening is often the only thing and the best thing you can do to help.

A lady always acknowledges a friend's loss, whether it's the big game or a beloved relative.

A lady doesn't ask the details of an accident or fatal illness; she just says she is sorry to hear of the loss.

A lady knows that when it comes to grief, just a few words mean a lot and if appropriate, a hug can say what words cannot.

Chapter 24

TELEPHONES AND MESSAGES

*E*ven when your parents deem it appropriate for you to have a cell phone, most families with children will still have a landline phone. Your older relatives probably have one too.

Your mom might have a funny story about the time when you were barely old enough to put a sentence together yet you answered the home phone and kept her boss on the line for five minutes, pleading, "Can you go get your mommy, please, and bring her to the phone?"

But that's only funny when a cute little toddler does it, and only once. Anyone who is old enough to answer the telephone should know how to use it properly.

That means how to answer a home phone, how to place a call, and how to take a message. Just because the person you are talking to can't see you doesn't mean you don't have to use good manners.

You do

Speak clearly and pleasantly when you answer.

You don't

Shout, mumble, or grumble into the phone.

Why

The caller should not feel as if his call is an imposition before he even states his purpose.

You do

Say either "Hello" or "Hello, this is the Taylor residence."

You don't

Say "Hey" or any other slang by way of greeting.

Why

Unless you have caller ID, you don't know who the caller is, and anything less formal than "Hello" does not make a favorable first impression.

You do

If the call is not for you, ask the person calling to hold for a moment while you quietly place the receiver down and get the person they are calling, or cover the phone while you summon that person.

You don't

Shout into the phone, "Mommmmm! It's for youuuuuuuuuuuu! It's Mrs. Adamsssss!"

Why

Mrs. Adams was not expecting someone to shout into the receiver and did not have time to move it away from her ear before you nearly ruptured her eardrum.

You do

Let the person who answers the telephone when you have placed a call know who you are.

You don't

Ignore their greeting and abruptly ask for your friend Paige. Or even worse, say "Who is this?" to the person who answers the phone.

Why

You wouldn't walk into someone's house without saying hello and announcing yourself. The way you announce yourself to the person answering the phone depends on who the person is. If it's your friend's father, you say, "Hello, Mr. Holmes. Is Paige available?" If it's your friend's brother, you can say, "Hi Travis. Is Paige at home?"

You do

Simply tell the caller that the person they are asking to speak with is not available; then ask if you may take a message.

You don't

Share that your parents are not at home or that your father is in the shower.

Why

It is not necessary to share that much specific information; it might even be unwise if you are home alone and the caller is a stranger.

You do

Write the caller's name and number on a message pad or clean sheet of paper, and place it where it will be found.

You don't

Write the message on your hand or a napkin or scribble it across the top of your little sister's drawing.

Why

The point of taking a message is to deliver information. No one would think to look at your hand, a napkin will likely be thrown away, and you'll be in big trouble if you ruin your sister's picture.

～

A lady asks permission if she needs to use the phone in someone else's home.

～

A lady returns the phone to its base and does not leave it wherever she last used it so the battery dies and no one can find it.

～

A lady does not chew gum, eat food, or drink beverages while on the phone.

～

A lady does not hang up on the person answering the phone if she has called a wrong number. She says, "I'm sorry to bother you. I have called the wrong number."

A lady does not call another person's home before 8:00 a.m. or after 8:00 p.m., unless it's very important.

～

A lady leaves a clear, short message on an answering machine, including her name, how she can be reached, and a brief reason for her call. She does not go on and on as if she is having a conversation.

～

A lady does not ask a caller what the nature of their call is.

～

A lady repeats back the caller's number just to be sure it's correct.

～

A lady does not scribble the caller's name and number. She writes the information legibly on a message pad so that it can be easily read.

Chapter 25

CELL PHONES: TALKING AND TEXTING

Few milestones in a young person's life are more eagerly anticipated by girls than the birthday that earns a cell phone. You might be ten or twelve or thirteen when your parents decide you are mature enough to have and take care of your own phone.

Even a kindergartner can figure out how to use a cell phone, but there's a big difference between knowing how to operate a cell phone correctly and how to use one with consideration for others.

Bad cell phone manners are not confined to tweens and teens; grown-ups who should know better do rude things with their phones all the time. Maybe it's because they didn't grow up with cell phones as a standard convenience of daily life.

But you did, which means that as soon as you are given the privilege of having your own cell phone, you should start practicing good cell phone manners.

You do

Know and observe the rules regarding the use of cell phones in school.

You don't

Try to sneak out a text from the phone in your lap or hidden behind a book.

Why

Besides disrupting the classroom, cell phones could easily be used for cheating on tests and assignments. There is no good reason to use a cell phone during class, and if you are caught, your phone could be confiscated by the teacher and not given back until your parents are informed, which is a good way to lose your cell phone privileges altogether.

You do

Lower your voice if you must use your phone in public.

You don't

Talk and laugh loudly on your phone in public places.

Why

Other people who don't know you and even those who do know you should not be subjected to a one-sided conversation that has nothing to do with them—particularly one that includes personal information or inappropriate language or comments.

There is no need to raise your voice when talking on a cell phone. If you are in a loud place, or the person you are calling is, move away from other people so that you can hear, or so you can raise your voice just enough to be heard. If that still doesn't work, tell the person on the other end of the line you will call them back.

You do

Turn your ringer off and put your phone in your purse or pocket in restaurants, church, synagogue, movie theaters, and any place where there is an audience.

You don't

Open your phone in a dark theater to check messages or send a text.

Why

Think of the racket if everyone left their phones on in a restaurant. A ringing phone interrupting a sermon, musician, actor, or dancer is disrespectful to that person and the rest of the audience. Opening your phone in a dark theater distracts everyone around you and breaks the magical spell cast in a darkened room.

You do

Finish your call or your text before ordering a sandwich at the sub shop or milk shake at the ice cream stand.

You don't

Continue talking on the phone or texting while the cashier or server is trying to do their job and conduct business with you.

Why

Talking on the phone while ordering a cheeseburger and fries may not only result in you getting a chili cheese dog with onion rings; it is the height of rudeness to treat someone in front of you as if they don't exist. Because this rude habit is so prevalent, many stores now post signs that say, "We will not wait on you if you are talking on your cell phone. Please hang up before reaching the counter."

You do

Answer your phone when your parents call.

You don't

Ignore your mom or dad calling because you're busy or having fun with your friends

Why

One of the reasons your parents got you a cell phone is that you are growing up and spending more time away from their watchful eyes. That doesn't mean they don't worry and won't want to check on you. Or maybe they have something important to tell you. As long as your parents are paying for your phone, answer their calls.

A lady does not interrupt a face-to-face conversation she is having with someone in order to take a call or read and reply to a text.

A lady does not bring her phone to the family dinner table.

A lady does not talk on the phone at the table in a restaurant, even a fast-food restaurant.

A lady does not take or place a call when she is a passenger in a car. If it is very important for her to check in with someone, she can say, "Do you mind if I take this quick call? It's my dad." Or she can send a very brief text.

A lady does not have an inappropriate ringtone.

A lady does not text while she is walking.

Chapter 26

THE COMPUTER

Among life-changing inventions, the computer ranks right up there with indoor plumbing and electricity.

Computers are a bit more complicated to use. It's simple to turn on a faucet or a light, and turn them off when you no longer need them. Turning on a computer is just the beginning. The most important thing to know is how to use it properly and safely.

When you were small, you probably used the family computer in a common area under an adult's supervision. As you got older, you gained more independence on the computer. You may have one of your own, or use the computers at your school or in the public library. That means you have more responsibility to operate the computer appropriately.

There are so many uses for the computer, you'll wonder how anyone—like your parents and grandparents—ever lived without them. You use it to research for an English project, or look up show times for the movie you and your friends want to see. You'll write papers, design PowerPoint presentations, and you might even create your own blog. You'll send e-mails, IM your friends, post on bulletin boards, and maybe participate in online forums and chat rooms.

At the same time, there are many opportunities for online misuse, abuse, and even downright risk to your safety and security.

Never lose sight of the fact that though your computer is an ingenious piece of technology, it connects you to real live people. And while it can bring the whole world to your fingertips, it can also take you to places you shouldn't and don't really want to go.

You do

Follow the rules for computer and Internet use that your parents, school, or public library set.

You don't

Try to skirt your way around security barriers, sneak onto inappropriate Web sites, or enter chat rooms clearly intended for older people.

Why

Like any tool, if used improperly, the Internet can cause you and others harm. Do not share your password with anyone except your parents if they request it for security purposes, and do not fill out any forms that ask for your personal information. Do not post your address or phone numbers on your Facebook profile, or send them in an e-mail. Do not download anything from a Web site you are not familiar with.

You do

Create an e-mail address that is appropriate for a young lady your age.

You don't

Create an e-mail address that is suggestive or in bad taste, or one that uses your full name.

Why

Think of the impression you want your e-mail address to make not just to your peers, but also to your family, teachers, coaches, a clergy member, or the parents of the child you babysit. Using your full name as your e-mail address, like laurenmariesmythe@ gmail.com, allows people you don't know to find you too easily.

You do

Carefully word your e-mails so as not to offend anyone.

You don't

Send an e-mail in anger or to avoid talking to someone face-to-face.

Why

E-mails lack the nuance and emotion of speech, and can easily be misunderstood and misinterpreted. Emoticons help, but seeing smiley or frown faces all over a text can get annoying. Keep your e-mails short and to the point, and read them over again before hitting the send button.

⁓

A lady doesn't use all uppercase letters for emphasis. IT MAKES IT SEEM LIKE YOU ARE SHOUTING, and a lady doesn't shout at others, even when she is angry or upset.

⁓

A lady doesn't say anything in an e-mail or on a public post that she would not say in person.

A lady never puts anything that could harm or hurt another person in a public forum like texts, e-mails, Twitter, or Facebook.

~

A lady doesn't think that because she can post a mean comment or ugly rumor on a blog anonymously or with a pseudonym, it's okay. If it were okay, a lady would not have to hide her identity.

~

A lady doesn't monopolize a computer used by others at home, at school, or in the library.

~

A lady should use hand sanitizer before and after typing on a public keyboard.

Chapter 27

USING SOCIAL NETWORKS

*F*acebook was launched in 2004 and has more than six hundred million users. If you're old enough and your parents gave their permission, you are probably one of them, along with nearly all your friends.

Chances are your friends' parents, your siblings, your aunts, uncles, cousins, and even your grandparents are also on Facebook. It's quite likely, even probable, that your teacher, principal, scout leader, coach, music instructor, minister, rabbi, and Sunday school teacher are too.

That doesn't mean they are all your Facebook friends. And that may make you think there is no way they will see the vulgar words you've used, the ugly gossip you participated in, the hurtful thing you

114

said about someone, the fib you told them, or the questionable photo you posted.

You would be wrong. No matter how high your privacy setting—and for your personal safety it should be set as high as possible—there is no such thing on the Internet as total secrecy. There is going to be some way that the people who hold you accountable, the people whose regard and respect you want, the people who trust you to do the right thing, the people who care for you the most, are going to see the thing you would not want them to see.

The possibility of getting caught by your parents or a teacher is not the reason you should not fib, use vulgar language, participate in name-calling or ugly gossip in a public forum, or post an inappropriate photo of yourself.

You should not be doing those things because they are wrong, they are hurtful, and they do not present you as the fine, mature, responsible, intelligent, thoughtful, and considerate young woman you are.

You do

Set your privacy settings to protect you and your family's safety.

You don't

Include your home address or telephone number on your information page.

Why

You do not want the millions of Facebook users to be able to see your profile, information, photos, and friends. People who are your close friends already know your address and telephone number. There is no good reason to make it available to everyone else.

You do

Respond in some way to friend requests.

You don't

Feel obligated to accept every friend request.

Why

Would you open your door to anyone who knocked and asked themselves in for dinner? Of course not. You are under no obligation to accept friend requests from people you hardly know, people you don't know at all, or people you do know and would not be friends with in real life. Simply hit the "not now" or "ignore" button. De-friending someone is okay too, as long as you don't post that you have done so on your wall for the rest of your friends to see.

You do

Know the difference between posting on a wall and sending a private message.

You don't

Post private things about you or your friends on a wall.

Why

If you post "Leila is so mean not to invite Cassie to her birthday party" on your wall, or "I'm sorry Leila was so mean to you" on Cassie's wall, all of your friends and all of Cassie's friends will be privy to something that should be between you and Cassie. Or between Cassie and Leila. When a thought or feeling or message is even remotely personal or private, send it to your friend through the message feature on Facebook.

You do

Share fun things and good news on your wall.

You don't

Share how ugly your big sister was to you, or that your brother failed his math test, or that you and your best friend had a huge fight.

Why

Facebook is called a "social network," not a "sibling revenge network," "family secrets network," or "group therapy network." Keep it light and do not share other people's behavior or status on your page.

You do

Create entertaining photo albums on your Facebook page of parties, family members, vacations, school events, and special occasions.

You don't

Include every single photo you have ever taken because you don't have the inclination to edit, or include or tag photos of people that are unflattering or might be embarrassing.

Why

Your friends will probably get weary of the album of your family trip to New York City at the eighty-seventh photo of an unidentified building taken from your taxi window. Then they will miss the really cool photo of you ice-skating at Rockefeller Center. It would be impractical to ask permission of every person in a group photo, but you should use your judgment in deciding which photos to post or tag.

A lady does not ask to friend someone more than once if there is no response to the first request.

⌒

A lady does not believe that having 874 "friends" means she is popular. It might mean she is indiscriminate.

⌒

A lady does not post or tag unflattering photos of her friends.

⌒

A lady does not create or join a "group" intended to hurt or degrade someone else, even if it isn't someone she knows.

⌒

A lady does not constantly update her status or send out a tweet to publicly document every moment of her day or every thought that crosses her mind.

A lady does not engage in Twitter wars. You can do a lot of damage in 140 characters.

A lady does not use inappropriate language on someone else's wall or when commenting on their status.

A lady knows that it is easy to put something on Facebook, but very difficult to remove it. Think before you post.

Chapter 28

TAKING
PHOTOGRAPHS

*T*hanks to the compact size, instant access, and simple operation of digital and cell phone cameras, there is very little that happens in young women's lives that can't be documented with the click of a tiny button.

Girls take pictures of their friends, their family, their pets, their cute shoes, their new dress, their dinner, their manicure, their birthday cake, and with an outstretched arm and steady hand, themselves.

And then they share—almost exclusively through social networking. It's fun, fast, and easy.

But it's not always appropriate or proper. Just as there are times to use your cell phone and times to put it away, there are occasions when photography is better left to a professional, or avoided entirely. Just as there are thoughts and comments we don't share with everyone, there are photos we don't share with everyone and photo opportunities we don't take advantage of just because they are there.

It is not wise or safe to take inappropriate photos of yourself to post on your Facebook page or send to anyone from your cell phone. Even when someone promises not to share a photo, once it is out of your hands, you relinquish control of that photo. Do you really want everyone in your school to see something that would embarrass you? If you receive a photo that makes you uncomfortable, you should delete it. If the person in the photo does not know the photo is being shared, you should find a way to let them know privately.

You do

Ask permission to take a photograph of a stranger or someone else's property.

You don't

Snap a photo of that adorable baby, that funny dog, or the great boots the girl at the next table is wearing.

Why

Even when people are out in public places, there is an expectation of at least a semblance of privacy and personal space. Invading that privacy and space is akin to walking into their home uninvited, or taking something that doesn't belong to you. Tell the baby's mother that her baby looks just like the little girl you babysit and ask if you can take her photo to show the little girl's mother. Tell the dog's owner, or the boots' owner, that you want a dog/boots just like theirs and ask if you can snap a quick photo.

You do

Take photos quickly if you are in a congested area.

You don't

Block foot traffic or someone's view, or monopolize the popular landmark while others are waiting.

Why

We all want well-composed and flattering photos, but planting your group in the middle of the sidewalk, or in front of spectators at the football game, or around the historic landmark while you check each shot until you get the perfect one isn't fair to others. In fact, it's annoying.

You do

Offer to take a photograph for strangers.

You don't

Impatiently tap your foot while they try to take their own couple or group photo.

Why

When you want to include everyone in a moment or a memory, aren't you grateful when a stranger steps up and offers to take the photo so everyone can be in it? It is a thoughtful gesture that is always appreciated.

You do

Take photographs of parties, family celebrations, sporting events, and casual get-togethers.

You don't

Take photographs during a wedding ceremony, baptism, confirmation, or bar or bat mitzvah, or during a live performance.

Why

Religious ceremonies are reverent occasions to be observed and witnessed with respect and regard for the participants. Most people hire a professional who knows how to be inconspicuous. Live performances before an audience require tremendous focus and concentration. The click of a camera or a flash of light is intrusive and distracting. Family and friends should take their photographs after the ceremony or performance.

A lady never takes a photograph of another person, even a stranger who is unaware of the photo, with the purpose of using it to make fun of that person.

⌒

A lady does not take photographs of people when they are asleep, or otherwise incapable of actively participating in the moment.

⌒

A lady does not share unflattering or inappropriate photographs of people— even if she is really, really mad at someone.

⌒

If a lady is unsure if posting a particular photo will offend or hurt someone, she asks permission first.

⌒

A lady does not post so many photos featuring herself as the sole subject that she appears to be self-obsessed and narcissistic.

TAKING PHOTOGRAPHS

Chapter 29

GOSSIPING AND KEEPING SECRETS

*S*haring information is a good thing to do when the information you are sharing is relevant, helpful, or important. If one of your soccer teammates needs a copy of the practice schedule, or a classmate misplaced the reading assignment, or you hear of a great sale on the running shoes that a friend loves, you share that information.

Gossip can be a fun and amusing interaction among friends when it is harmless and impersonal. But mean-spirited gossip and unfounded rumors can and often do have unforeseen consequences.

With the instantaneous capability of "sharing information" that texting, e-mailing, instant messaging, and social networking offers, the most unfounded rumors and ugly gossip can spread as fast as a wildfire and cause just as much damage.

Unless there is a very good reason for doing so, breaking a promise to keep a secret is a serious violation of the trust someone places in you.

You do

Have fun speculating with your friends about a story in a celebrity news magazine, what the stars wore on the MTV Awards, and if the leading actor and actress in your favorite television show are dating in real life.

You don't

Help spread rumors that your single English teacher is having a relationship with the married coach of the football team because they often have lunch together, that the girl running for class treasurer is a shoplifter, or that several members of the freshman football team are taking steroids.

Why

Spreading rumors that can cause lasting and sometimes irreparable damage to another person's reputation, their standing in their community, or their future is one of the worst things you can do morally, and you could also be held accountable by authorities for helping spread them.

You do

Keep a friend's secret if he or she confides in you.

You don't

Keep a secret if it involves the person doing harm to themselves or others.

Why

If your friend tearfully shares with you that her parents are talking about separating and possibly getting divorced, and asks you not to tell anyone, not even your parents, you don't. Your friend is counting on you to be a safe haven to share her sadness and anxiety. If your friend tells you more than once that the turmoil in her home is causing her to hurt herself or want to hurt herself, you should go to your parents, a teacher, or a guidance counselor and ask for their help in managing a secret that big.

You do

Consider if something you are hearing or saying about someone who is not present is something that would be said if she were.

You don't

Participate in gossip and talking about someone behind their back because everyone else is doing it, because you think it will never get back to the person, or because you think it will make you more popular to add fuel to the gossip bonfire.

Why

Gossip has a way of getting back to the person being gossiped about. Participating in gossip will not make you more popular, but walking away from it will gain you a reputation as a loyal friend and someone who "doesn't have a mean thing to say about anyone." That's the kind of reputation you want.

~

A lady doesn't tell one friend that another friend is talking about her behind her back; a lady speaks first to the friend spreading the gossip.

~

A lady doesn't tell things that another girl or boy did or said, or secrets they shared years ago that would be embarrassing to that person today.

Chapter 30

THE SLUMBER PARTY

A slumber party is a pretty funny name for a party where the point is basically not to slumber at all. The most successful slumber parties are the ones where the guests stay up all night eating, watching movies, doing each other's nails and hair, sampling beauty products, trying on clothes, taking lots of pictures, texting boys, playing music, and talking.

Any parent who has hosted a slumber party would add "squealing" to that list. There's nothing quite like the sound of six girls simultaneously emitting high-pitched squeals to make parents think they are in imminent danger of a tornado or under attack from an alien army.

Slumber parties can be the most fun thing in the world, but some guidelines of conduct can make the experience more enjoyable for you and your friends, and almost bearable for the host parents.

You do

Participate in all the activities with the other girls.

You don't

Sit in a corner and text another friend all night, or call home at one in the morning and beg someone to come get you.

Why

Things don't always go as we wished or anticipated. If you don't like the movie being shown, feel that you are being left out, or are not having a good time, make the most of it and remember that the party isn't for you, but for the birthday girl. In the morning when you wake up, you can make a private call to your mom or dad and ask to be picked up early. Or in sticking it out, you might discover you had a good time after all.

You do

Find the hostess's parents to say thank you and good-bye when your ride comes to pick you up.

You don't

Sneak out the door when your ride texts you to let you know they're outside and waiting.

Why

Thanking your friend is not enough. You must also thank your friend's parents, who put up with all the noise, lost a good night's sleep, and enjoyed none of the fun. Besides, if they don't see you leave, they might be concerned that you may have wandered off in the night.

You do

Bring things to share—a type of candy you know the birthday girl loves, fun colors of nail polish, individual packs of false eyelashes.

You don't

Bring only enough for you and the birthday girl, anything you couldn't bear to accidentally have broken, eye makeup to share, or glitter.

Why

A slumber party is a communal activity, so check before the party to see how many guests are expected so you know how much candy or how many packs of false eyelashes to bring. No matter how cute it looked sprinkled on that model in the magazine, glitter is never a good idea in real life, especially not in someone else's house.

⌒

A lady brings her own pillow, face wash, toothbrush, and toothpaste to a slumber party.

⌒

A lady doesn't leave anyone out.

⌒

A lady helps the hostess pick up in the morning.

⌒

A lady doesn't go anywhere in the host house except the area designated for the slumber party.

⌒

A lady does her best not to squeal after midnight.

Chapter 31

LOSING GRACIOUSLY

*T*he word *loser* has such an ugly sound to it. And as we all know, it feels even worse.

Losing feels bad, but it's nothing to be ashamed of if you did your best. In any contest or competition, there will be a winner and there will be someone or many someones who don't win.

You really can't win them all. No one can. Not even the University of Connecticut women's basketball team, who did win a record-setting ninety games in a row until December 30, 2010, when the University of Stanford Cardinals got the better of them. That made Stanford the winners. Did it make UConn losers? Technically yes. But did they act like losers? Did they stomp around and kick basketballs when they lost to the Cardinals? No. They shook the hands of every person and coach on the team that defeated them.

They might have cried in the locker room, but they were dignified in public.

Every year at the Oscars, there are five actresses who are nominated for Best Actress. Out of all the hundreds of actresses in hundreds of roles that year, just five are honored for their performances. And of those five, only one will win. Four will lose. Do any of the four losers open their mouths in disbelief, roll their eyes in disgust, or crumble in tears when their names are not called? Of course not. They smile and applaud their colleagues. Even if their heart is breaking with disappointment. They are actresses, after all.

Loser is an ugly word, but being ugly about losing is not going to make you feel any better. It will only succeed in making you look even worse than you already feel.

YOU DO

Congratulate the winner.

YOU DON'T

Burst into tears, run off in a huff, throw a hissy fit, or stomp your foot and cry "Unfair!"

Why

Calling attention to yourself in such a self-absorbed fashion takes away from the attention that the winner of the competition deserves. Losing won't reflect negatively on you. It's reacting poorly and immaturely that will hurt your reputation.

You do

Hold your head high even when you lose.

You don't

Walk around like a loser.

Why

If you did your best and tried your hardest, you have nothing to be ashamed of. Someone else ran faster that day, mastered a jump you hadn't quite perfected, or hit a note you somehow missed. Next time, you'll do better, but only if you believe you can.

A lady does not blame her loss on an unfair call or a judge favoring her competitor.

～

A lady does not blame her teammates when her team loses.

～

A lady concedes the spotlight to the winner.

～

A lady is dignified in defeat.

Chapter 32

IN AN AUDIENCE

*T*here will be times when you are a member of an audience for a performance you really want to see. Maybe it's a concert by a singer you're crazy about, or your best friend's performance in the *Nutcracker*.

There will also be times when you're forced to attend a lecture on "Teens and Technology" with your mom, or when your grandmother has decided to take you to the opera, whether you like it or not.

Though you are more likely to pay attention and be engaged with a performance that interests you than one you are sure is going to bore you to tears, being respectful to other members of the audience as well as the performers requires certain niceties and some traditional rules of conduct.

Movie theaters are more casual than performance

halls, and movie tickets aren't quite as expensive as those for plays and concerts, but disrupting or interfering with another audience member's enjoyment is thoughtless and rude, whether you are at the opera or in a movie theater.

You do

Arrive in time to get to your seat before the curtain goes up or a performance begins.

You don't

Walk down the aisle of a theater or performance hall while someone is singing, playing, or acting.

Why

Entrances are for performers, not audience members. If you arrive late, wait in the back of the theater until a break in the action or until an usher escorts you to your seat.

You do

Face the people you pass as you navigate the row to your seat, and say "excuse me" as you go.

You don't

Go down the row with your back to the people already

seated, or go so quickly they don't have time to move their knees, feet, purses, or water bottles.

Why

No one wants a rear end in their face, which is what they will get if you go down the aisle with your back to them. At the same time, do not press your rear end into the backs of the heads of the people in the row in front of you. Make yourself as small as possible and be aware of all your possessions as you go. If you step on someone's toes, say "I'm sorry." If you are already seated and someone needs to pass you by, rise enough so that your knees are out of their way.

You do

Sit still and attentively during the performance or lecture.

You don't

Fidget about, cross and uncross your legs, hit the back of the seat in front of you with your foot, or sigh loudly and repeatedly.

Why

Even if you have been forced to attend the concert, play, or lecture against your will, the other members of the audience want to be there. Your theatrics and squirming about draws their attention away from the stage and is disturbing to those around you.

A lady uses the restroom before entering the auditorium or during intermission.

A lady carries a lozenge of some type in her pocket or purse if she has a cough.

A lady does not rummage around in her purse, rustle her program, or chew gum loudly during the performance. In fact, chewing gum is best disposed of before a performance begins.

A lady does not hurt her host's feelings by showing her boredom or impatience.

A lady uses only one armrest and cup holder.

A lady turns off her cell phone or at least the ringtone before she enters any theater. She does not open her cell phone to check messages or text during a performance or a movie.

A lady follows the lead of the audience in applauding or standing if she is not sure what to do.

Chapter 33

ATTENDING A RELIGIOUS SERVICE

*I*f you attend religious services on a regular basis with your family, you already know what is expected of you. By now, you have graduated out of children's church and attend the entire service. There are probably times it seems so long and the sermon is so boring that you wish you were back in children's church. But you are growing up, and you should be proud that your parents and clergy consider you mature enough to be with the adults.

There will be times when you may be invited to attend church with a friend. While every denomination and religion has its own order of service and rituals, sometimes these even vary from one congregation to another.

Though it may not be familiar to you, there's no need to be nervous, even if your family doesn't regularly attend a church or synagogue and the only times you ever go are for holidays like Christmas, Easter, Rosh Hashanah, or Yom Kippur.

You should keep in mind that you are a guest in a house of worship and follow the basic rules that you would as a guest in the home of someone you are meeting for the first time. Watch what your friend does for guidance, and if you are unsure about something, ask.

You do

Ask your friend in advance what the proper dress is for her house of worship.

You don't

Assume that wearing your best clothes is the right thing to do.

Why

Some churches have become very casual, with blue jeans and sneakers the norm. If that is the case, you would feel uncomfortable in your best dress and heels. On the other hand, if you wear jeans and everyone else is dressed up, you'll feel disrespectful. Asking for guidance is the smart thing to do.

You do

Sit and stand when the rest of the congregation does.

You don't

Cross yourself or genuflect, join in the prayers, or take communion, unless it is part of your tradition.

Why

Following the lead of the congregation as they sit and stand is expected. If your faith does not make the sign of the cross or genuflect at the altar, you are not expected to fumble through it as a guest. If you have a fundamental disagreement with some tenet of this church's faith, you are not required to join in as others recite their creed, but you are expected to remain quiet and respectful as others do. There are some faiths that only offer communion to members of their own faith, and it would be awkward of you to presume that communion is open to all. If the worship leader announces that communion is open to all and you would like to participate, you may do so.

A lady does not bring anything to eat or drink, or chew gum, in the sanctuary.

⟳

A lady turns her cell phone off before entering the sanctuary.

⟳

A lady does not wear revealing or inappropriate clothing to religious services.

⟳

A lady does not bring a book to read during the service; she sits with good posture and is attentive.

⟳

A lady does not indicate she disagrees with the theology or doctrine of a particular faith during the service, even if she does. That is a conversation to have later at home with one's family.

Chapter 34

TRAVELING ON A PLANE

*O*f all the ways you can travel, flying on a plane is the most fun, exciting, and grown-up. It can also be a bit complicated.

It's not like hopping in the family car in your sweat pants and T-shirt with your pillow and iPod, when the biggest thing you have to worry about is making sure your brother doesn't cross the line onto your side of the backseat.

More than likely you'll be flying with your parents or another grown-up and they'll help you through, but there are some things to keep in mind to make the experience easier and more pleasant for you, your family, your fellow passengers, and the flight attendants.

These days, airlines pack a lot of people—and their belongings—into very limited, confined, and inflexible space, so it's very important to be considerate of others.

You do

Familiarize yourself with the basic rules of airport security.

You don't

Wear your lace-up boots, bring a quart-sized bottle of face wash, bury your laptop at the bottom of your carry-on, or make jokes about the sharp objects in your nail kit.

Why

Airport security is very serious business, and security personnel will not take kindly to jokes about safety infractions. Other passengers are anxious to get through the screening area as quickly as possible and if you have to unlace your boots and unload your bag, they will get irritated. Wear slip-on shoes, take your coat off, and have your laptop out of your bag before getting in line. And do not carry bottles of fluid more than three ounces in your carry-on bag. Everyone will be very impressed with your maturity and expertise.

You do

Go directly to your seat, hold your carry-on in front of you, keep your purse close to your body, and stash your things in the overheard bin above your seat or under the seat in front of you as quickly as possible.

You don't

Linger in the aisle, let your bag bump someone in the shoulder or head, or block traffic while you unload your book, laptop, and iPod from your backpack.

Why

Airlines need to get people seated and planes off the ground as quickly as possible. One person's cluelessness can affect an entire aircraft.

You do

Keep in mind that you will be seated in very close proximity to others.

You don't

Bring anything with a particularly strong scent—you or food—onto the plane, or wear something so scanty that the person beside you is disturbed or repelled.

Why

Odors—whether it is your new perfume or the jumbo bean burrito you bought before boarding—have nowhere to go on a plane except up the nostrils of the people close to you. Strong perfume can cause headaches. If you must bring food on the plane, make it something odorless and tidy. Skimpy tank tops and super-short miniskirts are not appropriate for air travel.

A lady follows the instructions of the flight attendant and does not press the call button unless it is very important.

A lady does not turn the volume up on her iPod or laptop so loud that other passengers can hear.

A lady does not recline her seat all the way, kick the seat in front of her, or grab it when she has to stand up.

A lady uses only the areas
assigned to her seat.

~

A lady brings something on the plane
to occupy herself with so she does not
annoy others.

~

A lady does not use the airplane's
restroom as a place to put on her makeup,
redo her hair, or spray on perfume.

Chapter 35

DRESSING APPROPRIATELY

*W*ouldn't it be embarrassing to show up at a pool party wearing a pair of shorts and a T-shirt over your bathing suit if everyone else was in party clothes? The invitation did say "pizza and swimming" but in hindsight, you should probably have erred on the side of caution, worn that cute sundress, and brought your bathing suit in a tote bag.

Sometimes we know exactly what type of attire is expected of us. Some schools require uniforms or have a strict dress code, and there's not much leeway permitted. When you're on a team, you know just what to wear to a game. If you play in a student orchestra, the dress code is probably pretty strict for girls and boys.

In other situations there are a lot of opportunities

to express yourself with your clothing, and as many opportunities to make a wrong choice. This is especially true at your age, when you're too old or big for lots of the clothes in the girl's department, and too young for many of the more grown-up clothes in the junior department. Advertising and media often show girls your age dressing ten years older than they really are. It's not always easy to figure it out.

That's when erring on the side of caution is not an error at all. Unless you are trying to call attention to yourself and provoke gossip—and why would a young lady do that?—it is a better choice to dress so that people don't remember exactly what you wore rather than have them whisper about your short skirt or your low-cut top. Good taste is always in style.

You do

Think about the message your outfit is sending and where you are sending it.

You don't

Wear your designer label clothing when you are volunteering in a homeless shelter or soup kitchen.

Why

Volunteering for people who have no food while you are wearing a pair of boots that cost the equivalent of a week's worth of groceries is insensitive and separates you from those you are serving.

You do

Have fun with fashion.

You don't

Load up on every trend the minute it hits the stores.

Why

Unless you have an unlimited clothing budget, a closet full of this season's trends has a very limited style life. For example, don't buy three pairs of the cropped cargo pants and four pairs of the skinny jeans all over the fashion magazines for fall; buy one of each, and use the money you saved for some cool new tops.

A lady does not wear clothes that are too suggestive or excessively revealing, no matter how proud she is of her figure.

~

A lady who wears a short skirt remembers she is wearing a short skirt and walks, sits, reaches, bends down, and climbs stairs accordingly.

~

A lady does not wear stained or torn clothing out of the house.

~

A lady does not wear clothing that is too small.

~

A lady does not wear T-shirts printed with vulgar, obscene, or suggestive language or images.

~

A lady knows that a basic white blouse, dark skirt, and classic cardigan in her wardrobe will take her anywhere.

Chapter 36

COSMETICS

Convincing your parents that you're old enough to start wearing makeup might be hard.

There is no "right" age for makeup, other than the age you and your parents agree on, but most girls start using simple cosmetics sometime around sixth or seventh grade.

Your makeup should not lead your face into a room. Cosmetics are intended to enhance a woman's assets and beauty, not construct a mask.

For young girls taking their first plunge into the wonderful world of cosmetics, a natural look is preferable and will probably be the most acceptable to parents. That means no raccoon eyeliner, no line of foundation on your jawbone, no garish streaks of pink blush on your cheekbones, no purple lipstick, and no baby-blue eye shadow from lid to brow.

Only the luckiest teens in the world make it through adolescence without suffering at least an occasional breakout on their faces or other parts of their bodies. Even more important than what color eye shadow you wear or what kind of mascara you choose is to start taking care of your skin at an early age and adjusting the care as your skin changes. That means keeping it clean and using the right products for your skin type and problem areas.

You do

Take care of your skin, keeping it as clean as possible. It's the only face you've got, and you'll be living in it for a lifetime.

You don't

Pop or pick at pimples; put new makeup on top of old makeup; wear heavy makeup when participating in sports or at the beach or pool; or go to bed with makeup on, no matter how tired you are.

Why

A dirty face with clogged pores is a breeding ground for skin trouble. Popping and picking at pimples is so tempting, and may be a quick fix, but will most likely cause scarring. There are plenty of better options available, and if over-the-counter products are not working, ask your parents if you can see a dermatologist. Makeup that streaks as a result of sweating or heat is not attractive or good for your skin.

You do

Go with your mom or girlfriends to a department store for a consultation and free application with a professional who represents a line of cosmetics suitable for young women.

You don't

Go to the drugstore and buy multiple shades of foundation, eye shadow, blush, and lip gloss to take home and find the ones that work.

Why

Makeup in department stores is more expensive than makeup in drugstores, but if a professional helps you find exactly the right shades and applications for your skin type, you can actually save money, and learn how to use them properly.

You do

Share makeup tips with your friends.

You don't

Share makeup with your friends, especially any product that goes on your eyes.

Why

    Pink can be a fun shade of eye shadow. Pinkeye is not fun. It is extremely contagious, and sharing eye shadow, eyeliner, and mascara can result in sharing much more than you intended.

      ∿

A lady always removes her makeup and washes her face before bed.

      ∿

A lady does not apply makeup in public.

A lady is careful when trying on clothes that she does not stain them with her makeup.

A lady keeps her cosmetics and skin care products in a case, not scattered all over the vanity in the bathroom she shares with her siblings.

A lady wears sunscreen every day; otherwise she will look like an old lady long before her time.

Chapter 37

FRAGRANCE

*A*side from stinky diapers, babies have the most delicious smell. Which is why you always see grown-ups—especially moms and grandmoms—lean in toward babies with their noses, inhaling deeply as if smelling a loaf of bread or a bouquet of flowers.

There's really not much distinction between the smell of girl babies and boy babies, or girl toddlers and boy toddlers, or even seven-year-old girls and seven-year-old boys.

That changes about the time kids hit double digits. Boys start to smell like sweat, pepperoni pizza, locker rooms, and sporty body spray. Girls start to smell like fruit and flowers. Everything from body lotion and bath gel to lip gloss and even deodorant smells like green apples, raspberries, freesia, strawberries, lilac, pineapple, roses, and grapefruit. Slumber parties smell like an entire orchard and as if a garden has burst into bloom overnight in the hostess's bedroom.

As you get older, you'll leave behind a trail of empty fruity bubble bath bottles and begin experimenting with cologne and perfume. There are thousands of scents to choose from and a few things to remember before dousing yourself with a bottle of Happy, Princess, or Daisy.

There is a difference in strengths and prices of fragrance. The least expensive and lightest scent—and a good choice for young ladies—is eau de cologne or eau de toilette.

You do

Test perfume by spraying lightly on the inside of your wrist and wait at least thirty seconds to sniff, then sniff again in about thirty minutes when it has time to interact with your body's chemistry.

You don't

Smell a perfume insert in a magazine or on someone else and decide that's the one for you, just because you love it.

Why

Scent interacts differently on every body.

What smells lightly floral on your friend might be nauseatingly sweet on you.

You do

Lightly spray or dab cologne on your pulse points— inside of the wrist, behind your ears, and in the crook of your knee.

You don't

Spray cologne all over your body.

Why

Cologne is not a spray tan. You should wear your scent; your scent should not wear you.

You do

Keep in mind that when it comes to fragrance, less is more.

You don't

Wear so much perfume that people two feet away from you can smell you coming, or that your perfume hovers in a room, in a car, or on the furniture for hours after you've left.

Why

Scent should be elusive and fleeting, not an assault on the senses. If your scent is so strong that others can not only smell it but also taste it, you are wearing far too much.

⌇

A lady does not wear heavy fragrances when she will be in confined spaces like a car, a plane, or a movie theater.

⌇

A lady does not reapply perfume like lip gloss. Fragrance lingers long after *you* no longer smell it.

⌇

A lady does not wear a heavy scent to breakfast unless she wants to give her parents a headache.

⌇

If a lady accidentally applies too much cologne, she uses a baby wipe or hand sanitizer to lessen the impact.

Chapter 38

PERSONAL GROOMING

When you were younger, personal grooming was as simple and quick as taking a shower once a day, washing your hair when it got dirty, and brushing your teeth in the morning and before bed at night. When you were going out to play with your friends, you just got dressed; if you had long hair, you probably pulled it up in a ponytail.

Those days are as much a part of your past as *Sesame Street* and Barbie dolls. Now, your little brother complains about your stuff all over the bathroom you share, your mom is tapping her foot outside your bedroom door while you change clothes five times before school, and your dad just shakes his head and wonders where his "little girl" went.

At your age, getting ready to go out takes a lot longer, and requires a lot more stuff and steps. That's a natural part of adolescence, but young ladies are mindful that their stuff and their personal grooming habits don't impose on other people's space or time.

You do

Keep your face, body, and hair products in one area in a bathroom that you share.

You don't

Scatter your things all over the vanity and tub.

Why

Bathrooms are contained spaces with limited shelf space. If you take more than your share, you're not sharing at all; you're hogging. You might keep all your products in a waterproof plastic basket you can put out of sight in a linen closet or your bedroom when you are not using them.

You do

Talk to a grown-up before coloring your hair or piercing anything.

You don't

Come home from the mall with pierced ears or emerge from the bathroom with platinum blonde hair and say "Surprise!"

Why

Piercings and hair coloring are dramatic changes and not easily reversed should you decide that, for now, you're not that interested in wearing earrings every day, or that platinum blonde isn't really your color. An adult will point out that spontaneous actions can have long-term consequences.

A lady clears the drain in the shower after she washes her hair.

A lady does not shave her legs in the sink.

A lady styles her hair, puts on her makeup, and applies body products behind closed doors in her bathroom or bedroom.

A lady does not try to shape her eyebrows herself, but asks for professional help.

A lady removes or applies nail polish in her bedroom or bathroom, and never in a common space where the smell would overwhelm everyone.

Chapter 39

MANAGING
A PERSONAL
EMERGENCY

*P*ersonal emergencies aren't things like floods or earthquakes or tornadoes or hurricanes. Those are major events with tragic consequences.

Personal emergencies are not life threatening or even dangerous. They may even seem silly in comparison to real emergencies. A stuck zipper or broken bra strap is nothing compared to actual disasters. But when they happen to you, at that moment it's unsettling and upsetting.

Accidents happen. Being prepared for unexpected snafus doesn't make them go away, but does make them easier to manage.

You do

Blot a splash of spaghetti sauce or salsa that has landed on your white blouse.

You don't

Rub at it frantically with a napkin and water trying to get it out.

Why

Rubbing at something that has the potential to stain will only work it into the fabric and guarantee it will never come out. As hard as it is to be patient, just gently blot up what you can, and get the garment to a professional as soon as possible—whether that's your mom or the dry cleaner.

You do

Pin a few safety pins to the lining of your purse or keep them in the change pocket of your wallet.

You don't

Use a stapler to close a split in the backside seam of your jeans, or use Scotch tape for a torn hem.

Why

Why do you think they call them safety pins?

Safety pins are perfect for temporary repairs on rips, torn straps, hems, and broken zippers. Staples can scratch and tape won't hold. If you have some safety pins in your purse when a friend's adorable sundress pops a strap on the way into the party, you will be a hero.

You do

Prepare before leaving the house when it's your time of the month.

You don't

Leave the house without extra feminine hygiene products.

Why

If you are having your period, it's not the best time of the month to wear your white slacks or yellow dress. Why tempt fate? If you are close to starting or are on your period, you must carry tampons or sanitary pads in your purse. If you get your period unexpectedly when you are away from home and none of your friends can help, a thick layer of toilet paper will work as a panty liner until you can find the product you need. If you should stain your clothes and you have a sweater or a jacket, or can borrow one from a friend, wrap it around your waist until you can get home.

A lady discreetly tells her friend if she has spinach in her teeth, a crucial button undone, or needs a breath mint. She expects her friends to do the same for her and will not take offense.

⌒

A lady takes off both shoes if one breaks, and doesn't hop around on one foot.

⌒

A lady always carries her identification, a bit of cash, and a bank card if she has one.

⌒

If a lady has a serious allergy to any medication or food item, she carries the proper notification.

Chapter 40

SITTING

*I*f you're big enough and old enough that your feet hit the ground when you're sitting in a chair, then you're big enough and old enough to mind how you sit.

We don't mean the procedure that takes you from standing to being seated. (Other than not plopping down so hard on a chair its legs quiver, there's not much to it.)

Once you are actually seated, however, there are a few things you'll want to get in the habit of doing. They might feel unnatural at first, but before long you won't even think about them.

You do

Keep your knees together.

You don't

Spread out on a seat as if you're trying to use up all the space.

Why

Sitting with your legs spread wide when you are wearing a dress might show your underwear. Since that's not what you want to do, keep your knees less than an inch apart when you're wearing a skirt or dress. Sitting pretty is keeping your knees together even when you're wearing jeans, pants, shorts, or sweats.

You do

Cross your legs at the ankles.

You don't

Cross your legs at the knees.

Why

Etiquette classes for young ladies teach that crossing one leg over another is considered very unladylike. Many etiquette rules have been relaxed for our more casual lifestyle, but there are still times when it is more appropriate to cross ankles rather than knees, particularly in spaces with limited leg room, such as airplanes and theaters. It's easy to do: once you are seated with your knees together, slant your legs so your knees face one corner of your chair, then cross the opposite ankle over the other. For example, if you slant your legs so your knees point left, cross the right ankle over your left.

～

A lady doesn't slump in her chair; she sits up straight.

～

A lady doesn't tip her chair back.

～

A lady doesn't put her feet on the top of the chair in front of her.

～

A lady doesn't sit cross-legged on the floor unless she is wearing pants or shorts.

～

A lady in a short skirt pulls the hem down as she is sitting.

Chapter 41

WALKING

*I*t's a walk in the park" is an expression people use to describe something that is really easy. Walking seems so simple; it's just one foot in front of the other.

Walking gracefully takes a little more awareness and effort. Not that you should emulate runway models; they don't walk that way off the runway.

Walking with grace puts good posture in motion. Your shoulders are level, your spine is straight, your head is up, your heel hits the ground first, and the weight rolls to the ball of your foot, which you use to push off for your next step. Your gait is natural— not tiptoe tiny and not as if you are preparing to do the long jump. Back in the previous century, young women used to practice walking properly by balancing a book on their heads as they walked back and forth across a room. That probably seems a bit extreme these days, though it might be fun to see how you do.

When you walk with grace and confidence, you present yourself as a positive person. Knowing how is the foundation for mastering a skill unique to women: walking gracefully and confidently in high heels.

You do

Buy shoes in the correct size.

You don't

Buy shoes that are too small thinking they will "stretch" or shoes that are too big thinking you can make them work.

Why

Shoes that pinch or rub will make you hobble. Shoes that are too big make you look like a little girl trying on your mom's shoes. Neither scenario is pretty. No matter how cute the shoes are, if they're not available in your size, they're not the shoes for you.

You do

Practice walking in heels at home before going out in public.

You don't

Think your first pair of heels will not require some practice.

Why

When you learned to ride a bike, you started with something your size equipped with training wheels. Think of heels the same way; start with something small and low to the ground. Every time you gain height in the heel, practice walking around at home on the carpet, hard surfaces, and especially the stairs. There's little that looks as awkward as tripping over your own feet or wobbling and falling off your heels.

A lady doesn't shuffle as if she's sweeping the floor with her shoes, but picks up her feet when she walks.

⌐

A lady doesn't walk so heavily that she sounds like she's wearing horseshoes.

⌐

A lady doesn't wobble on her heels; if you do, you need more practice.

⌐

A lady doesn't swing her bottom from side to side when she walks.

Chapter 42

ENTERING AND EXITING A CAR

*W*atching a bunch of little kids get in and out of cars is like watching a litter of puppies climbing over each other trying to get to their mother. Up until recently, your biggest concern about getting into a car was scrambling ahead of your siblings so you didn't have to take the middle, or sitting next to your best friend so you could share the earbuds on your iPod.

Now that you're getting older, your bigger concern is getting into and out of a car gracefully. When you are wearing a dress or a skirt, particularly a short dress or skirt, it is important to know how to do it without flopping and heaving, or even worse, showing your underwear.

To avoid that, follow these simple steps for getting into a car.

1. Back into the car or enter sideways, bottom first onto the seat.
2. Once your bottom is on the seat, with knees together, swivel your legs into the car.
3. If you have to slide over to make room for another passenger, place your hands flat on either side of you, slightly lift and swivel your bottom in the direction you need to go, then follow with your legs, knees together.

To get out of a car without showing everyone what color underwear you are wearing:

1. Pull down your skirt as far as it will go.
2. When the door is open, with knees together put your legs out first and onto the ground if you can reach; if you're in a Texas-sized pickup truck or SUV that has a running board, place both feet there.
3. Place your hands on the seat on either side of your hips and push yourself up and out. If there is a built-in handle on one side of the car interior, use that to pull yourself up while using your other hand as leverage to push yourself up.

YOU DO

Accept a hand when it is offered to help you out of a car.

You don't

Swat the hand away saying, "Do I look like an old lady to you?"

Why

Offering someone a hand to get out of a car, particularly when the car is either very low to the ground or very high off the ground, is a thoughtful thing to do and has nothing to do with your age. But reacting rudely will reflect on your maturity.

A lady does not scramble headfirst into a
car or crawl across the seat to get out.

～

A lady always wears her seatbelt, even if it
will wrinkle her clothes.

～

A lady does not get into a car with an
impaired driver.

～

A lady does not bend over with her
bottom in the air to get something she
left in the car, but gets back in the car
to retrieve it.

Chapter 43

HELP WITH YOUR COAT AND OTHER SMALL COURTESIES

As you enter a more grown-up social world, with any luck you will encounter gentlemen who have been taught by their mothers and fathers to practice certain courtesies toward women. A young man who has been taught these things is lucky indeed; good manners are one of the most valuable assets anyone—boy or girl—offers the world around them.

When courtesies are offered, you accept and say "thank you," even if you don't think you need the help that is being offered. To refuse a gesture of good manners is bad manners.

When someone opens a door for you, you say

"thank you." When someone offers to share his or her umbrella in an unexpected downpour, you say "thank you." When someone pulls out your chair in a restaurant, you say "thank you."

It's important to know how to accept certain courtesies. Walking through an open door is easy. Knowing how to be helped with your coat is a little trickier.

Presumably, the person who offers to help with your coat knows what to do: he stands behind you, holding your coat open at waist level, with the arms of the coat lined up with your arms. You hold your arms straight and slightly behind you, insert both hands into the arms of your coat, and let him pull it up to your shoulders until you can grasp the front of your coat with your hands.

If a gentleman or a server in a restaurant or a banquet pulls out your chair for you to sit at the table, stand with your back to the chair until the back of your knees hit the chair's seat. Slowly lower yourself at the same time the chair is being pushed in. If you are still too far from the table, rise slightly so that the chair can be nudged forward a bit. If you are offered help to get up from the table, lift your bottom up slightly from the chair so it can be slowly pulled backward, then stand, being careful not to knock the table.

You do

Check your coat at a restaurant or banquet hall if a coat checkroom is available and is offered to you.

You don't

Hang your coat over the back of your chair so that the servers and other diners trip on it.

Why

Would you bring your coat to the table at home? At nicer restaurants and for formal occasions, coat checkrooms are provided as a courtesy to you, other guests, and staff. Check your coat, as well as umbrellas, scarves, gloves, and any bags you might be carrying. You do not check your purse. Be prepared to tip at least two dollars when retrieving your belongings.

If a checkroom is not provided, a lady folds her coat over the back of her chair or puts it in the corner of a booth so it is out of the way and not in foot traffic.

⌒

A lady always carries some money in her purse and does not rely on the generosity of others.

⌒

If her purse is very small, a lady puts it in her lap or on the floor under her chair. She does not put it on the table, hang it on the back of her chair, or leave it anywhere someone might trip over it.

⌒

A lady says "thank you" when someone opens a door for her, helps with her coat, or helps with her chair.

Chapter 44

RESPONDING TO INVITATIONS

Invitations are kind of like presents. They're fun to receive and open, and they're almost always in celebration of a special occasion. Some you like better than others, but all of them require a response of some kind.

When you were little, invitations to birthday parties or July Fourth cookouts probably came to your parents, especially if it was something to which your whole family was invited. Your mom or dad answered for everyone, and you all went as a unit.

As you got older, invitations came directly to you, and though you still need to ask your parents' permission to attend or check to make sure there isn't something else on the family calendar, responding to invitations is increasingly your responsibility. That means you need to learn how to do it correctly.

Some invitations might be face-to-face, very casual, and have nothing to do with a birthday or celebration. Maybe after softball practice Thursday afternoon Ellie says, "Hey Katie, I'm having the team over to swim Saturday after the game. Bring your suit if you can come." Your teammate isn't expecting you to call her on the phone to confirm, but even if you end up not going, at the game you tell her you won't be able to attend, and thank her for the invitation.

Other invitations are more formal, like ones that come in the mail or via Evite. In these instances, the hostess would like to have an idea beforehand of how many guests to expect.

Being invited to something doesn't mean you are required to accept. You might have a previous obligation, or you might not have seen the person throwing the party since fourth grade and would feel awkward going to a party where you don't think you'll know the other guests.

You do not have to explain or make up an excuse. But you do have to respond. "Thank you for asking. I'm sorry I can't make it" is absolutely enough.

There are two types of "formal" invitations—regrets only and RSVP.

You do

Let the hostess know you cannot attend if the invitation says "regrets only."

You don't

Call to let the hostess know you will be attending.

Why

When an invitation says "regrets only," it is usually for something like a come-and-go open house. Or maybe it's an end-of-the-season team party where the hostess expects that the entire team will be attending. If you cannot attend, you send your regrets.

You do

Reply either way to an invitation marked RSVP. (French students may know the acronym is for *répondez s'il vous plaît*, which literally translated means "respond if you please." It may be easier to remember as "please respond.") Be sure to respond before the deadline.

You don't

Wait so long to reply that the hostess or her parent has to call you on the phone to be sure you received the invitation.

Why

The invitations that ask for an RSVP are the parties for which the hostess needs to know in advance how many guests to expect. It might be a skating party or a bowling party. Maybe the hostess is planning to take her guests to see a concert or a play and her parents need to know how many tickets to buy. Maybe the party is at a restaurant and they need to know how large a table to reserve. If you forget to reply and show up anyway, it is bound to cause a problem. The easiest thing to do is reply as soon as you get the invitation and after you check with your parents.

A lady does not put off replying to an invitation in case something "better" comes along.

A lady does not accept an invitation and then cancel at the last minute for a party she thinks will be more fun.

A lady does not change her no to a yes at the last minute because something she thought would be more fun did not materialize.

If a lady gets ill or a family emergency arises that prevents her from attending a party where she is expected, she calls the hostess as soon as possible. She does not ask another guest who is going to let the hostess know, or count on her hostess checking her e-mail before the party begins.

Chapter 45

WOULD YOU LIKE TO DANCE?

At some point in your life, sooner than you may think, you will be confronted with an invitation to dance. With a boy. It might be the seventh-grade mixer, your best friend's bat mitzvah, or ninth-grade homecoming. Whichever one it is, the first time is the scariest.

The good news is, learning how to dance isn't that hard, especially if you do it with your friends. One day your mother may come to you and say with great enthusiasm, "I've signed you up for Fortnightly!" or "I've signed you up for cotillion!" If you have an older sibling, or friends with older siblings, you might already be familiar with the concept: a series of classes designed to teach young girls and boys the basics of dancing, social skills, and good manners in social situations.

At least, that's the theory. Fortnightly and cotillion classes are typically held every other week. There are rules about attire: girls wear dresses or skirts of modest length, boys wear coats and tie, and everyone wears dress shoes.

The instructor will put boys on one side of an imaginary line down the center of the room and girls on the other. At the instructor's signal, the girls and boys meet in the middle and the fun begins!

You might think that sounds like the worst idea imaginable. What if you stumble? What if you step on your partner's toes? What if your hands are sweating? What if you have to touch that awful boy who's been so mean to you?

Remember this: classes last for an hour to ninety minutes and anyone can endure anything for that long. It's not torture, it's the fox-trot. All fifty of you are in the same boat and worried about the same things. Everyone will stumble a bit and step on someone's toes, but everyone is so worried about what *they* will do wrong, they don't care what you're doing wrong.

You may not think you will ever in your whole life have reason to know the box step, the waltz, or the fox-trot, and certainly not the cha-cha. But ten years down the road when you're a bridesmaid at your cousin's wedding and the cute groomsman asks you to dance, and the band inexplicably kicks off a cha-cha, you'll be glad you are not still the awkward young girl at her first Fortnightly class, with no idea where to place her hands or put her feet.

You will not need to know how to waltz or cha-cha at your school dances. On the rare occasions that boys and girls dance together in seventh and eighth grades, it's usually more freestyle. You do need to know how to respond if a boy should be brave enough to approach you among your friends and ask you to step onto the dance floor with him.

You do

Accept an offer to dance when one is extended.

You don't

Dismiss the invitation with a curt no.

Why

It takes a lot of courage to walk across a room to ask a young woman to dance; don't make him feel like an idiot for taking that chance. An invitation to dance is not a proposal, and accepting doesn't mean you're going steady.

You do

Pay attention to your partner while you are dancing.

You don't

Look over his shoulder at someone else or talk to your friend dancing beside you.

Why

For the duration of the dance, you and your partner are a duo. When it comes to dancing, three's a crowd.

You do

Accept his apology graciously if he steps on your foot.

You don't

Make a big deal and end the dance.

Why

Stepping on a partner's toes happens to even the best dancers and for all you know, your foot might have been in the wrong place.

You do

Understand that formal dancing requires touching.

You don't

Act as if your partner has a contagious disease and hold yourself at arm's length.

Why

You can't dance the waltz or the box step without touching certain neutral parts of your partner's body, and vice versa. If your partner tries to pull you too close or places his hands inappropriately and you feel uncomfortable or threatened, you should pull discreetly away and say you would rather not finish the dance.

If a lady has not had any formal dance instruction, she should ask one of her parents or a friend for some pointers before attending an event that might involve dancing.

A lady lets the gentleman take the lead, even if she is the better dancer.

A lady doesn't say, "I'm a terrible dancer" as she is being led to the floor.

A lady says, "Thank you for the dance" when it is over, and is free to return to her seat.

⁓

A lady is not required to stay on the floor with her dance partner for a second dance.

Chapter 46

THE DATING GAME

*D*ating is even more daunting than dancing, especially since a date lasts a lot longer than a dance. Sometime in middle school, girls and boys start to spend more time together in coed groups. Sometime in middle school, girls and boys start to use social media or texting to "talk" to one another outside of the group.

And sometime in middle school, a boy—one you like as a friend, one you "like-like," or one you have never noticed before—might ask you on a "date." It could be as simple as a suggestion you meet at the movie, or maybe something more involved, like going to that seventh-grade mixer. First dates make everyone nervous, no matter how old they are, but even more so when you have no experience at all. When someone asks you for a date, it is helpful to have some idea of how to respond so no one's feelings get hurt.

If it's someone you "like-like," you simply say "sure." If it's someone you know you like only as a friend but you're afraid he is hoping for more, try to steer it back to something casual, maybe by suggesting that you get a group together.

If it's someone you know you don't like at all, you need to be honest because you don't want to lead him on. Don't go on and on with all the reasons you can't. Simply say, "Thank you, but it's not really a good time."

If the boy is someone in your class or a friend of a friend, but you don't know him well, there's nothing wrong with giving it a chance, as long as the proposed date is something you feel comfortable with. You never want to put yourself in a risky situation for the sake of a date, or go anywhere with a boy without letting your parents know.

You do

Thoughtfully respond to an invitation from a boy.

You don't

Say "are you kidding?"

Why

Whether "are you kidding?" means "oh wow, I never thought you'd ask!" or "no way, not in a million years!" the most likely response you will get to "are you kidding?" is "yes, I am" and a hasty retreat.

You do

Say you have to ask your parents, especially if you want some time to think about it. At your age, you more than likely do have to ask your parents.

You don't

Say you have to ask your parents and then never get back to the boy.

Why

It's rude to leave someone hanging on and wondering. If your parents say no, let the boy know right away. If you're not comfortable with a one-on-one meeting, it's better just to be honest.

You do

Tell the truth, taking into account how hard it is for a boy to ask for a date.

You don't

Make up a lie about your sick aunt or having to babysit your little sister.

Why

Lying is never a good idea or the proper response under any circumstance. Inevitably, if you say you can't go bowling with him because you have to take care of your sick aunt, you will run into him at the mall. That would be very awkward.

~

A lady doesn't say unkind things to her friends about a boy she has turned down for a date.

~

A lady doesn't post on her Facebook page how dorky her eighth-grade mixer date was dressed or how boring her homecoming date was.

~

A lady doesn't text or call others when she is on a date.

A lady says "thank you" at the end of the evening, even if she did not have the best time.

⌒

A lady can discreetly call her parents if she finds herself in a situation that is uncomfortable to her, or involves doing something she is not allowed to do.

Chapter 47

BEING A CONSIDERATE HOUSEGUEST

*A*s you're growing up and are more independent, you'll probably have invitations to spend a few days at someone's house. Your friend might invite you to come to her family's lake house or mountain cabin for the weekend. Your parents might go on a vacation and make arrangements for you to stay with your aunt and uncle or with a family friend.

Being a houseguest is a little different from spending the night or attending a slumber party at your friend's house. The stay is longer, which means you'll need to adapt to your host's habits and routine, while also being mindful of the regimen of the house you are visiting.

You do

Bring a small token of appreciation with you to give when you arrive.

You don't

Arrive lugging only your suitcase or purchase an expensive or unsuitable appreciation gift.

Why

Bringing something everyone can enjoy always makes a good impression. A loaf of good bread or a box of homemade cookies for everyone is thoughtful, and something your mother or father can help you with. An expensive piece of pottery is unnecessary and a DVD of a movie that is too mature for every member of the family is not suitable.

You do

Follow the routine of the household.

You don't

Sleep in until noon if everyone else gets up at eight, expect breakfast when everyone else is having lunch, or stay up watching television alone in the den hours after everyone else has gone to bed.

Why

Your hosts have already gone out of their way to make you comfortable; don't disrupt their household in return. It is your responsibility as a houseguest to blend in with the order of the home.

You do

Make your bed in the morning, pick up your room, and keep all of your bath and beauty products in a toiletry bag.

You don't

Bring along sloppy habits from home, leave your things lying about in common areas, leave a clump of hair in the tub drain, or wipe your eye makeup off on the hand towel in the bathroom.

Why

You are not in a hotel with housekeeping service; you are a guest in someone's home and should keep the space you are using as neat as you found it. Be sure to bring your own eye makeup remover, hair care products, toothbrush, and toothpaste.

A lady doesn't use her host's phone or computer without permission.

A lady doesn't take anything from her host's refrigerator or pantry without it being offered first or unless she's been given blanket access.

⌒

A lady doesn't monopolize a bathroom she is sharing with someone else.

⌒

A lady always brings a robe to wear over her sleep clothes and to the shower.

⌒

A lady offers to help at mealtime, take out the trash, or pick up the popcorn from the floor in the family room after movie night.

⌒

A lady asks her host if she can strip her bed the morning of her departure.

⌒

A lady writes a thank-you note as soon as possible after her visit.

Chapter 48

BEING A GOOD HOSTESS

*B*eing a hostess can mean anything from asking a friend to come home with you after school to study, to a sleepover with your three best friends, or an end-of-the-season party in your basement for your entire basketball team.

The bigger the guest list and the more moving parts there are to the event, the more things you have to prepare for and think about. You don't have to have the most food, the best assortment of beverages, the latest state-of-the-art multimedia system, or the biggest house to be a good hostess. The most important part of being a good hostess is making your guests welcome when they arrive and comfortable while they are there. Most of all, you want them to leave feeling that they had a wonderful time.

You do

Introduce guests who don't know each other.

You don't

Assume that people will introduce themselves.

Why

Jenny might say to Sally, "Hi, I'm Jenny," but she isn't likely to offer the information that she knows you from the swim team. It's your responsibility as the one person in the room who knows everyone to make introductions and connections. You would say, "Sally, this is Jenny. We have been on the swim team together at Seven Hills since we were six. Sally goes to St. Cecilia with me." Give guests who don't know one another conversation starters.

You do

Put anything away that you or your parents could not bear to see broken.

You don't

Make a guest feel terrible if they break a plate or spill grape soda on the white rug.

Why

Accidents happen, so you don't want to take a chance on your mother's favorite piece of Italian blown glass getting knocked off the table and ending up on the floor in a million pieces. Check the room before your guests arrive and put precious items away or on a higher shelf. If a guest accidentally drops a plate or drips soda, they already feel embarrassed. It's your duty as a hostess to make them feel better, not worse.

You do

Consider who is on your guest list.

You don't

Plan the party with only your own likes in mind.

Why

Just because the only kind of soda you drink is root beer, doesn't mean all of your guests like root beer. In fact, some of your guests might hate root beer. Pepperoni pizza may be your favorite, but there may be someone at your party who loathes pepperoni. A Ping-Pong tournament is a lot of fun for everyone except the person who couldn't hit a Ping-Pong ball with a paddle the size of a hubcap. Have a variety of beverages, foods, and activities on hand so no one gets left out.

A lady greets and says good-bye
to every guest.

～

A lady spends a few minutes
with each guest.

～

A lady always offers her guest something
to drink, even if the guest is her friend
who lives next door.

～

A lady never eats in front of guests
without offering to share.

～

A lady doesn't share with others an
accident a guest in her home had.

Chapter 49

BOUNDARIES

When you were little, you needed help taking a bath, washing your hair, and getting dressed. Now that you're older, you can do all those things yourself, and you definitely want to do them behind a closed door.

When your mother, your sister, or your close friends want to tell you something privately, they might get very close to you so they can whisper it near your ear, and that's fine. But if someone you don't know very well or at all does the same thing, it's not fine. In fact, it probably makes you very uncomfortable.

Everyone has a need for boundaries, privacy, and personal space. You have the responsibility to respect others' space and every right to expect it for yourself as well.

You do

Knock on a closed door and wait for a response.

You don't

Knock and then barge in, or even worse, not knock at all.

Why

The door to a room might be closed because someone is changing clothes or using the bathroom. If you don't knock first and then wait until the person inside says "come in" or "just a minute," you might both be embarrassed.

You do

Ask your family to knock when your bedroom door is closed.

You don't

Turn your music up so loud when you're in your bedroom that you can't hear when someone knocks or calls your name.

Why

Privacy is different from isolation. If you are always locked in your room with your music turned up so loud you can't hear anything on the other side of your door, your family will begin to wonder why you are isolating yourself from the rest of the household, and they would have every right to be concerned.

You do

Set boundaries in the bedroom you share with your sister.

You don't

Leave your things all over her bed, desk, or dresser—or throw her things all over the floor if she leaves them on *your* bed, desk, or dresser.

Why

Sharing a room isn't easy, even if you and your sister are the best of friends. Setting boundaries and even an imaginary dividing line might sound silly, but knowing what the rules are in advance will help avoid and resolve issues in the future.

A lady doesn't slam a door.

A lady doesn't wiggle the handle of a
locked bathroom door to show the person
inside she's in a hurry. If the person in
the bathroom is taking a long time, a
lady softly knocks on the door and hopes
that is enough to let the person using the
bathroom know someone is waiting.

A lady doesn't go through other people's
things, read someone else's mail or
journal, or eavesdrop on a private
conversation.

Chapter 50

HELPING OTHERS

*I*t's human nature to help other people. It feels good to do a good deed, make someone smile, hear a "thank you," or get a pat on the back.

When you were little, your mom and dad may have taught you the importance of helping by asking you to "help" with dinner or "help" in the yard, even though you were so little it would probably have been easier for them to do it themselves.

If volunteering is something you have always done with your family, you know how rewarding it is, and that it helps you see that people are more alike than different. Volunteering is also a great way to make friends with people you would normally never meet otherwise.

As you get older, your help really makes an important contribution to your family and among

216

your friends, and can make a real difference in daily life, in your community, and even in the world.

There are many ways, big and small, to help others. Here are some small things that can make a big impact:

- Carry the grocery bags into the house for your mom without her having to ask.
- Donate the toys and clothing you've outgrown to a family shelter instead of throwing them away.
- Recycle.
- Read to the kindergartners in the aftercare program at school.
- Take your little brother to the park so your parents can go for a walk together.
- Write a letter to a member of the military.
- Sweep the porch for your grandparents.
- Pay a stranger a compliment.
- Lend a friend a listening ear.

When you take the initiative to help others, you show that you are growing up to be a fine young lady and an overall good human being.

You do

Answer a request for help affirmatively and cheerfully unless there is a very good reason you cannot.

You don't

Slam dishes down if your mother's request to set the table interrupts your phone call or television show, or kick balls around the garage if your dad asks you to put away all the sports equipment.

Why

Do you really need to be reminded how much your parents have done for you since even before you were born? Your mother would probably be agreeable if you asked permission to set the table as soon as the show is over, as long as you keep your word.

You do

Offer assistance to people with physical challenges.

You don't

Insist on helping if they decline your offer.

Why

Just as you would open and hold the door for anyone, you would offer the same courtesy to someone who is blind or in a wheelchair. You do not need to push the wheelchair or lead the blind person through the door. If they are in need of further assistance they will let you know how you can help.

A lady does not make her parents
ask twice for help.

A lady does not let other people down.

A lady puts herself in other people's shoes.

A lady helps even when no one will
know she has.

A lady does not keep a scorecard of
helpful things she has done.

A lady knows that helping others is
its own reward.

ABOUT THE AUTHORS

KAY WEST has been a professional writer in Nashville, Tennessee, for 30 years. She was restaurant critic for the *Nashville Scene* for 15 years and remains a contributing feature writer. She is Nashville stringer for *People*. She has written four books, including *How to Raise a Lady* and *How to Raise a Gentleman*, and co-authored *Dani's Story: A Journey From Neglect to Love*. She has raised a well-mannered daughter and a well-mannered son and is an avid baseball fan.

JOHN BRIDGES, author of *How to Be a Gentleman*, is also the coauthor, with Bryan Curtis, of seven other volumes in the best-selling GentleManners series. He is a frequent guest on television and radio news programs, always championing gentlemanly behavior in modern society. Bridges has appeared on the *Today Show*, the Discovery Channel, and *CBS Sunday Morning*, and has been profiled in *People* magazine and the *New York Times*.

Bryan Curtis is an author and the president of Dance Floor Books. He is the author/coauthor and editor of more than fifteen books, including the popular GentleManners series.

INDEX

D

E

F

invitations
    from boy, 200
    to dance, 193–198
    responding to, 188–192

K

knives, 61

L

licking fingers, 57–58
lies, 201
lipstick, 59
listening, 95
    to adults, 46–49
losing graciously, 134–137

M

makeup, 44, 156–160
messages from phone calls, 97–102
mistakes, apology for, 26–29
movie theaters, 138–139

N

nail polish, 168
napkin, 56–59
"no" as answer when asking permission, 36

O

odors, 150
overflattering, 53

P

parents, introducing friends to, 17
passing food around table, 52
performance, being part of audience, 138–142
perfume, 150, 162–164
period, planning for, 171
permission, asking, 34–37
personal emergencies, 168–172
personal grooming, 165–168
personal information, in introductions, 18

U

underwear, 44
uppercase letters, in e-mail, 112
utensils, 61, 64

V

vegetarian, 68
volunteering, 216–219
    clothes for, 153

W

walking, 176–183
water glass, 62
wrapping gifts, 80